HEADS UP

HEADS UP

Increase your sexual confidence, expand your sexual repertoire, and get the real low down on oral sex

Dr Teesha Morgan

Constance Lynn Hummel, MA

www.HeadsUpBook.com

Book cover and interior design by Marie Poulin.

Heads Up: Increase your sexual confidence, expand your sexual repertoire and get the real low down on oral sex / Dr. Teesha Morgan & Constance Lynn Hummel, MA. —1st ed.

ISBN 978-1-5141142-5-4

CONTENTS

Preface with Thanks

We decided to embark on this writing endeavour after we noticed a serious lack of reliable and up to date — yet light-hearted and interesting — resources we could recommend to our clients. We envisioned a book that combined extensive and diverse tips and techniques regarding fellatio, while still looking at the psychological and therapeutic side that may be blocking people from fully embracing or enjoying this type of intimacy. What we didn't take into account was the endless behind the scenes work required to bring this idea to life.

We could have never completed this book if it weren't for the help of a few key people who generously offered their time and skills in order to help make this project a success. Thank you does not begin to cover the gratitude we have for the people listed below.

Thank you Harrison for your patience and artful computer skills. You have helped us more times than we can count.

Thank you Marie for your amazing and creative design skills. Brilliance is too light a word when referring to you and your craft.

Emmy, your eagle eye, and editorial ability are amazing. Thank you for taking the time to read, and re-read, every draft we threw your way.

Uzma, what can we say? Thank you for the painstaking hours you put into doing our initial edits. You are an incredibly talented writer and editor, and we are so very grateful for all the work you put into this project.

Dan, you have been a mentor and friend who has guided us through the writing process. Thank you for your honesty, your editing expertise, and the hours you put into formatting our work.

Disclaimer and Other Legal Jargon

Good sex will not fix a bad relationship.

Now say it again.

Good sex will NOT fix a bad relationship.

In fact, good sex within a bad relationship will most likely drag it out, making it that much harder to leave.

What do we mean by a bad relationship?

Any relationship or encounter that repeatedly leaves you feeling disrespected, judged, dismissed, silenced, hurt (either emotionally, or physically), or devalued.

Any relationship in which you feel pressured to do things that you are uncomfortable with, that go against your values, or make you feel as though your boundaries are not being respected.

Sex and intimacy can be fun and playful, passionate and erotic, and sometimes even a bit weird and awkward. However, it should never leave you feeling hurt or ashamed of yourself or your actions. If you feel this is happening, first talk to your partner, then if things don't change, *run*—do not walk—away. We promise you, having better sex within these relationships will not help your cause.

That being said, good sex could help an otherwise healthy relationship that's struggling to feel stronger and more connected, or allow an already good relationship to become unbelievably great. Our goal with this book, however, is not to provide an exhaustive step-by-step guide to what you should be doing, but rather to get your imagination flowing to create possibilities.

No two lovers like the same thing. What creates toe-curling bliss for one may be irritating, painful, unpleasant, or just plain boring for another. Every mutually joyful intimate act is a co-creation between you and your partner(s). Talk to them, check in with yourself, and always make an effort to try new things. If it feels good, and you and your partner(s) are into it — you're doing it right.

Now before we get to the juicy stuff, we should also mention that a few sex acts we speak of may be illegal in some parts of the world. Please use your own discretion, know your country's laws surrounding sex and sexual acts, and continue at your own risk. We will not be liable or responsible to any individual or entity for any injury, ailment, loss, harm, or damage caused directly or indirectly by the information (or lack of information) contained within this book.

Although we have tried our best, this book is not perfect, nor is it intended to be the final authority on sex and sexuality. There may be moments during your reading when you find you disagree with us, are confused, offended, or even angry. These may be good times to reach out to a physician, therapist, best friend, or another support network. We realize what we present may not be for everyone, or applicable to everyone. Ultimately it is your life and your body: venture within the bounds of your common sense, at your own risk.

PART ONE: HEADS UP

1

Penises and How to Play With Them

Throughout our many years of research within this field, we have discovered that there are a number of excellent books written on sex. However, not all pass the test of time. The collective of written works are merely an expression of our time and culture; there are no Ten Commandments for great oral sex that we can throw your way. That being said, we will describe for you the dimensions of oral sex that often go unspoken. The need for these conversations is what our many years of clinical work and sexuality-based research have brought to our awareness. In this book we aim to provide positive sex talk for the sexually savvy, while inspiring jaw-dropping moments, and techniques that will blow your mind, for both amateurs and experts alike. So sit back, put your feet up, and get ready to laugh, explore, and get sideswiped by a few "Shut the front door!" moments.

The Definition

So, what does the word 'fellatio' actually mean? Simply put, it is the art of using your mouth to pleasure and stimulate a penis. The word fellatio comes from the Latin past participle of the verb fellāre, meaning to suck; the use of the term "blow job" to refer to fellatio is, therefore, quite ironic, as you'd be wise to channel a vacuum over a leaf blower any day.

Now although this Wikipedia® generated definition may give you an idea of what fellatio is, this definition may be a bit misleading, and lacks many crucial ingredients. Nowhere does it include the terms "amazing", "connecting", "incredible", "mind-blowing", or just plain "fun" to precede the term fellatio, and without those you're both missing out on all that oral sex has to offer. We would, therefore, like to encourage you to redefine fellatio as the artful choreographed collaboration of your mouth, your hands, your eyes, your chest, your tongue, your throat, your vocal cords, and even your sexually driven prowess, to stimulate your partner's penis, and surrounding sexually intimate areas, in ways that you and they find utterly sensational.

Now, if creating this titillating oral sex experience is of interest to you, we invite you to steal a few moments from your day to read these tips and tricks and see what works for you. We feel it's an investment worth making, because once you get your partner hitting those "Oh Oh Canada's," there's no telling where this orgasm related patriotism will take you.

DID YOU KNOW?

The echidna (an odd animal that looks like a cross between a hedgehog and an anteater) has a four headed penis. When the male echidna has sex with a female, one side of the penis seems to shut down, leaving only two out of the four heads in use. However the next time the male mates, the heads on the other side of the penis will be used. The female echidna's reproductive tract has two canals, therefore all four penis heads could not be active and grow in size.

2

Slang and Other Dirty Terms

You may question why such a fine and upstanding book would have a section on slang and dirty words — it is simply to inform you about the terms used in popular culture, and to encourage you

DID YOU KNOW?

Most male birds lack a penis. The Argentine lake duck, however, has a spiny member that measures upwards of approximately 17 inches, or around the length of its entire body. The penis is also equipped with a tip like a brush. This strangely shaped object is believed to help each drake latch onto an unwilling female, and brush out another male's sperm before injecting his own.

to think. Whether you feel intrigued, perplexed, or amused by the terms is a moot point.

FELLATIO AND ITS MANY FACES

- The Lewinski
- Playing the Skin Flute
- Smoking Pole
- Giving a Hummer
- A Blow Job
- A Bee-J (BJ)
- Giving Head
- Going Down
- Penile Tonsil Hockey
- Speaking into the Mike
- Polishing the Knob
- Meeting with Mr. One-Eye
- Playing the Pink Oboe
- Going Downtown
- Gamahuche
- Addressing the Court
- Blowing the Horn
- Milking the Yogurt Cannon
- Getting Protein Through The Meat Straw

3

Back in the Day

A Brief History and Background of the Penis-to-Mouth Relationship

The exact origins of fellatio may never be known. Historical references in text or imagery cross numerous societies and countless generations, but the precise location and time of its inception is beyond the scope of what we currently know. Therefore we offer here mere tidbits of its appearance across a few cultures and timeframes.

The Kama Sutra (or the Kama Sutra of Vatsyayana) was written in India no later than the fifth century AD. Kama Sutra means "love guide" and is best known for its detailed description of many penile-vaginal based sex positions; however it also includes several chapters on foreplay (which give instructions on embracing, kissing, touching, slapping, scratching, biting and sucking). The Kama Sutra covers fellatio in considerable detail, but only speaks of cunnilingus (a female receiving oral sex) briefly and barely mentions anal sex.

For more information on the Kama Sutra's recommendations see the Appendix section under Anatomy: Knowing Your Instrument.

Jumping centuries forward (into a more Western-based history), fellatio perks up its head in written text in the early 1800's. During this time, medical experts claimed that oral sex was an unnatural act because a female could not become pregnant from it. However, oral sex was present in pornography (photos and written erotica), where it was sometimes referred to as "gamahuching". Unlike today, a man in the 1800's who wanted some oral love, had to seek out a brothel with a girl who had a reputation for providing it. The code words to look for included the word "French", such as French-house or French talents, or women who named themselves after these code words, such as "French Marie". If he found one of these lovely ladies, he was usually safe to request oral sex.

In the New Orleans's red-light district, there was a famous brothel called Diana and Norma's. This was a French house with a fellatio specialty; in fact, their fellatio talents were so special, that's all they offered. Since oral sex was all there was to be had on the menu, Diana and Norma's took advantage of economics by becoming efficient interior designers and increasing turnover.

By building smaller rooms (as there was no need for beds) and increasing their turnover — as men no longer needed to take the time to fully undress — they were able to maintain a thriving business based solely on oral sex.

The most famous "fellationista" (yes, we just made up a word) was a lady by the name of Emma Johnson, often referred to as the "Parisian Queen of America." She had such amazing oral sex skills that she offered a "sixty-second plan." If any man was able to last longer than a minute without ejaculating, Emma gave her titillating talent away for free, not charging a penny for the blow job.

Attitudes towards fellatio, from the far East to the far West, have changed and evolved throughout the centuries and will most likely continue to do so as societies' behaviours change and adapt to what is considered "normal" for the time. All we can hope is that this evolution involves open communication, consent, and actions that help to perpetuate pleasure and love.

DID YOU KNOW?

The American Social Health Association began conducting surveys of the types of sexual acts that were requested of prostitutes in 1933. According to their stats, a mere 10% of requests made at this time were for sexual acts other than intercourse. However, by the end of the 1960's, 90% of the requests made were for oral sex, or a combination of oral and intercourse.

4

Before Your Oral Presentation: Outlook is Everything

Three important things to consider:

1. IT'S ALL ABOUT THE ATTITUDE.

Picture this: you are starving, you haven't eaten in weeks and someone offers you a large warm wiener schnitzel. You are so excited to devour this that your eyes grow large, you sink to your knees in anticipation, and you give it the kind of pleasure-filled excitement that only a ravenous individual could.

This mind-set can be what makes or breaks pleasurable oral sex. In fact, one might go as far as to say that attitude is 80% of what you need to master. Treating a penis like it is the best gift you have ever gotten is the best gift you can give, which brings us to our next point.

2. TO GIVE IS TO GET

The 1972 American pornographic film Deep Throat was one of the most popular and highest grossing films of its kind for good reason. It follows a young woman's journey to achieve an orgasm, discovering—through the help of her doctor—that her clitoris was actually located in her throat, causing her to have mind-blowing orgasms by giving fellatio. So how does this movie plot apply to you? Well, you can use it as a theoretical guide; most people think that by giving a blow job they are actually giving their partner something, i.e. the gift of pleasure. And although they are inherently right, you will do both yourself and your partner a great service by switching this thought pattern into believing that you are actually getting pleasure from giving them head. This switch in outlook may skyrocket you and your partner to a whole new level of horniness.

DID YOU KNOW?

Approximately 70% of heterosexual-identified females and approximately 85% of heterosexual-identified males have reported sexually fantasizing about oral-genital sex. We were unable to find similar research for homosexual-identified individuals.

3.   THE SHIFTING OF THE POWER DYNAMICS

Many believe that the very act of giving head is in some way submissive and degrading, and that this subservient role is not meant to be enjoyed. Now, we could write many pages exploring these beliefs and getting to the heart of where these feelings arise from and why they are blocking some from sharing the pleasures of oral sex; however we will not be exploring that here. You will find more about this in the second half of the book. For now, let's just break this down plainly and simply:

You have your partner's penis in your mouth. This organ is considered by many to be their most vital and precious body part. You, therefore, have the power to give immense pleasure. Your partner is in the most vulnerable position they can possible be in. They are actually submissive to you. As long as you are participating of your own free will—you run the show. The end.

5

Setting the Stage

Using Your Partners Sense of Smell to Your Advantage

According to research published in the Journal of Sexual Medicine, the correlation between sexual arousal, brain activation, and olfactory stimulation (our sense of smell) is paramount. Many individuals experience "strong" sexual arousal when their nose picks up a certain scent. In fact, feminine perfume produces the activation of very specific brain areas in males, and certain foods actually work to increase penile blood flow. For example, the chart below highlights the top 10 odours which produced the greatest increase in penile blood flow (according to the Smell and Taste Treatment and Research Foundation in Chicago).

Note: This may only be representative of a North American male-identified population given where the research took place.

INCREASE IN PENILE BLOOD FLOW PRODUCED BY TOP 10 ODOURS

Odour or odour combination	Average Increase
Lavender and pumpkin pie	40%
Doughnut & black licorice	31.5%
Pumpkin pie & doughnut	20%
Orange	19.5%
Lavender & doughnut	18%
Black licorice and cola	13%
Black licorice	13%
Doughnut & cola	12.5%
Lily of the valley	11%
Buttered popcorn	9%

Now it should be noted that the sample size was small – so don't fret if the scent of a doughnut doesn't get the penile juices flowing. The doctors concluded that the most effective scent was a lavender/pumpkin pie mixture; however, the results did depend on other factors, such as whether the participants' partners wore cologne and how many times they had intercourse in the last month.

In short, the only reliable conclusion to be drawn from this is that all sorts of smells—not just perfume or pumpkin pie—can increase penile blood flow or stimulate a male's brain function. Depending on the gentleman's age, he may also react differently to certain smells. For instance, older males tended to respond more strongly to vanilla.

So what does all this information have to do with you and why should you care? Well, it's basically insinuating that if you spray your sheets with lavender, have a pumpkin pie cooking in the oven, and dab a little vanilla behind your ear, you might just have to do a little less work when trying to get your partner hard.

OK, that may be oversimplifying things. The take home message is that smells can and do affect erections. Use this knowledge as you will.

"Anybody who believes that the way to a man's heart is through his stomach flunked geography" – Robert Byrne

THE SWEET SMELL OF SUCCESS, OR THE STENCH OF FAILURE

On the flip side of the penile arousal coin, nothing can kill the mood faster than offensive smells. This goes for you and your partner. You may want to suggest a pre-game shower to set the mood. You can playfully use this time to wash each other while allowing you both to move forward without the worry of coming face-to-face with unseemly smells. That being said, if your partner's smell is truly a barrier to you feeling comfortable and they are not willing to step up and take care of the situation with some gentle nudges, it is fair to explain that this is a large deterrent for you and that you both need to look for some ways that this can be addressed without hurtful comments or mood-killing put downs.

LANDSCAPING: IT'S NOT JUST FOR NATURE LOVERS

Everyone has their own preferences for the hair-down-there. Some people prefer a clean slate, some prefer a thoughtfully trimmed presentation, and others find perfection in letting it grow like nature intended—wild and free. Once again, if you find that your partner's preference in personal pubic expression is putting out your fire, maybe suggest trimming things up on their behalf as a "trust exercise" or a playful "I'll do you if you do me" activity in the shower.

LUBE (BECAUSE WETTER IS USUALLY BETTER)

Although many find that their saliva is more than enough, there are those occasional times when you need just a little more help. Adding a few drops of lubricant to your routine will allow for ease of slide and can take the pressure off if you're experiencing a bit of dry mouth. Using pre-cum for extra glide is helpful, but sometimes bedside lubricants are that extra aid to help things flow smoothly. Certain lubricants can also add a touch of delicious flavouring to enhance your oral sex giving experience.

The two most common types of personal lubricants are water-based and silicone-based:

Water-based lubricant doesn't break down materials found in condoms or sex toys, won't stain your sheets, and washes off easily. The downside however is that it isn't as slippery as, and dries out much faster than, silicone-based lubes. Therefore, you may need to re-apply often, as over time it evaporates and can leave behind a "pilling" effect.

Silicone lubricants are longer lasting, more slippery, can be used in water, and do not cause bacterial infections. The downside is that although these lubricants are generally compatible with condoms, they may not be compatible with certain sex toys, so it's important to double check the labels before using them. Also, since silicone-based lubes can be used in water, it takes a little more effort to clean up the aftermath of a generously applied lube-aided session, and it's very difficult to get out of your clothes and sheets. Additionally, from a taste/ texture perspective, silicone is not always the most appealing product to have in your mouth. However, silicone-based lube is an incredible aid when looking to perform an amazing hand job as it just keeps going and going, with no need for a reapplication.

Oil-Based /Petroleum lubricants such as baby oil, petroleum jelly, or massage oils will damage latex products and destroy your condoms. They may also lead to bacterial infections if used internally so the rule of thumb is that these types of lubricants are great for massages and outer-course (foreplay focused outside your orifices) but are not to be used with insertion of any kind.

Warming or cooling lubricants have additives that do just what the name implies: they give a cooling or warming sensation when applied to the skin. Some require you to blow on them to get the sensation kick started. Others require some type of friction to become activated. Many folks find the sensations to be a welcome additive, heightening the experience and their body's reaction. However, a quick word to the wise: be sure to start sparingly—and add more lubricant later if needed—as some of these products can pack a punch and no one wants to end their intimate evening with a panicked run to the shower to sooth a painful penis. For newcomers who may be using these lubricants for the first time, it is suggested to 'test-run' a new lube prior to engaging in vigorous sexual activity to ensure you and your partner both know what to expect.

Flavoured edible lubricants come in a variety of flavours and can come in handy for those who get a bit squeamish about the taste of a penis. In fact, many individuals don't enjoy their partner's natural taste, but don't mind giving oral sex when their partner's penis tastes more like a chocolate covered banana split. Using these types of lubricants can also be a fun way to spice up your routine by trying flavourings that really make you hungry for, and enjoy, oral sex.

Desensitizing lubricants work to minimize the sensations the penis is receiving; however, they are not recommended for oral sex as they will also desensitize or numb your mouth in the process. Not only that, they usually have a horrible taste. You may want to leave this type of lube in the nightstand until after oral sex, as it does have amazing benefits for helping to extend the length of penetrative sex.

TIPS FOR THE LUBE SAVVY

Some people don't like using condoms as they feel like they are losing the "true" oral sensation when there is a barrier in place. To help counter this feeling, place a few drops of lubricant inside the head of the condom before placing it over their penis. If your partner wants a little more added stimulation, use a cooling or warming lubricant.

It is recommended that oral sex occurring outside of a trusting committed relationship should involve condom usage to add an extra layer of safety. To help make the process of using protection more appealing, you may want to try putting on the condom with your mouth, not your hands (See Chapter 9 - Advanced Techniques to learn how to put on a condom with your mouth). To minimize the condom taste, use flavoured lubricant for this process.

When reaching for your bottle of lube, you should keep in mind that your lubricant—straight from the bottle—is not going to be warmed to a comfortable body temperature; therefore, you may want to place a few drops in your hands first before applying directly onto a sensitive body part. This will give you a chance to rub your hands together and warm up the lube to the desired temperature rather than shocking your partner with the touch of cool liquid.

Although many view lubricant as simply an aid for helping with penile glide, others have realized that lubricated testicles can also provide positive stimulation. Adding lube to the underside of the penis can help with perineal and testicle massages, which is a wonderful way to step up your oral sex activities (See Chapter 9 - Advanced Techniques for how to give a perineal massage).

"Courage /n./ Two cannibals having oral sex."
– Unknown

6

The BJ Basics

TEETH

It's not rocket science. As a general rule, most people with penises prefer that you keep your teeth away from their precious parts. That being said, some light nibbles through the underwear or the occasional playful and daring soft squeeze can be fun, but tread lightly...very lightly. Always be sure to check with your partner before adding gentle bites.

SPIT

The more the better. Don't try to swallow your saliva, let gravity take it down the shaft and aid in lubricating the penis. If you're having trouble getting enough oral lubrication, pop a mint in your mouth to get the juices flowing. Also, pre-cum is nature's way of helping out—let it lend a hand to improve your glide.

HANDS

Nature provided you with nimble fingers and opposable thumbs for a reason. Using one or both of your hands can be a helpful way of providing more stimulation, unless of course bondage and/or power play is at work, and then by all means, let your tongue aid where your hands cannot. Generally, most people report that they enjoy at least one hand on the shaft, exploring the testicles, anus or other sexually stimulating areas (nipples, thighs, frenulum, perineum, etc.).

TESTICLES

You may think they aren't part of "the job", but many people report that the testis will feel neglected if you pretend they aren't important. Using your hands, tongue, and mouth to engulf the testis is an essential part of foreplay, and the first step towards exploring the wonderful world of perineum and anal pleasure, if you so desire. Many individuals would find it difficult to ejaculate if you focused most of your time on this region; however, incorporating them into your routine, in some capacity, is something to explore.

SUCTION

Generally, you don't have to suck, or form a suction cup, after each stride up and down the shaft. Still, throwing in the occasional sucking behaviour—or sucking on release (when your mouth leaves the penis)—could be fun.

TONGUE

If attitude is the most important factor to giving great head, tongue and hand movements are a close second. Think of your tongue as a third hand, or an extra appendage to work into the mix. It can make its own trips up and down the shaft or spend some quality time on the corona. It's that gentle lick to add extra lube, that quick flicking motion to stimulate the frenulum, that tease to tickle the balls or inner thigh—it's an all-around self-lubricating pleasure giver. Use it each time, every time. Whether it's venturing out on its own or adding extra sensation while inside your mouth as you move up and down the shaft. For more specific 'tongue tricks' check out *Chapter 8 - Tips and Techniques.*

When/if your tongue gets tired and you need a break feel free to remove the penis from your mouth at any time and grab it firmly with your hand. Then lightly—or more aggressively

DID YOU KNOW?

Pre-cum is a made up of a secretion from the Cowper (bulbourethral glands) and urethral or periurethral (or Littre, named after Alexis Littre) glands. The prostate gland manufactures a portion of the next wave of secretions, which accounts for approximately 15-30% of the total volume of ejaculate. Followed by the testes, which contribute a very small amount of sperm (approximately 1% of the total volume of the ejaculate), and finally the seminal vesicles, which produce between 65-80% of male's ejaculate.

depending on your partners pleasure buttons—tap or smack the head of the penis against your lips . Some males find this facial tapping a nice interlude from suction lubricated pleasure.

THE SWITCH UP

Sometimes a motion that is done over and over again can get boring, lead to chaffing, turn a body part numb, or simply loose its edge. You may want to switch up your speed, direction, pressure, and type of touch. Repetitive motions up and down the shaft (whether with one's hand or mouth—or both) can produce an orgasm and ejaculation in many individuals; however, if you constantly begin and end with the finale, it can have adverse effects.

TO SPIT OR SWALLOW

No one can tell you what is best or "right". That is based on individual choice and preference. Many people feel that the conclusion to a fantastic blow job is finishing in their partner's mouth. Others couldn't care less. Some love to watch their ejaculate shoot, some don't ejaculate at all. This is something you need to discuss with your partner (to discover what they prefer) and is something you need to ask yourself in regards to what you're comfortable with.

ORGASM/EJACULATION CONNECTION

In most cases, an orgasm goes hand-in-hand with an ejaculation, but these two functions do not have to be combined as an orgasm can occur without the expulsion of any ejaculate. Some individuals can control the release of their ejaculate until they see fit, which may be after two or more orgasms.

LENGTH OF TIME

There is no allotted amount of time that you should be giving oral sex. Many like it quick and dirty; others enjoy the tease and find pleasure in making their partners beg for the release. Some males will last only a few moments, others never ejaculate from receiving oral sex. Long story short, it differs for every person and every occasion, as long as your partner is enjoying themself, and you're enjoying yourself (and you haven't gotten lockjaw or a hand cramp), then the length time is a not important.

RECIPROCATION

Reciprocation is not a must. It is however important that you and your partner are both OK with whatever arrangement you have discussed. If you don't enjoy receiving or giving that's OK, but the willingness of both you and your partner to reciprocate— or discuss why you are uncomfortable reciprocating—is what is important.

DID YOU KNOW?

The total volume of ejaculate is approximately 1-2 teaspoons (between 2-10ml). Semen volumes are affected by the amount of time that has passed since the previous ejaculation (with larger volumes seen after greater durations of abstinence from ejaculation). Semen contains, on average, around 15 calories, or less than one-tenth of a candy bar. Each milliliter of semen contains 50-150 million sperm, and a normal ejaculate contains between 100-700 million sperm however sperm account for less than 1% of the total volume of ejaculate.

COMING PREPARED

If you have long locks, or bang fly-aways, you may want to have a hair tie or clip on hand. A hair tie can also be used as a sexual aid, similar to pearls for a mid-show intermission. However, if you are fine with things getting a little messy—after all, that's what they made showers for—leaving your hair down can offer some fun options. For more tips on what you can do with your long locks, check out the Advanced Techniques Section.

CONDOM COURTESY

It is highly recommended to use condoms when having sex outside of a trusting committed relationship. While some believe condoms are only necessary for intercourse, the truth is that many STI's (sexually transmitted infections— formally known as STD's) can be passed from one person to another via oral sex. Now we will spare you the gory details and specifics in this section; nonetheless, we do encourage you to use protection when going down on your partner. To reduce stress and anxiety around condom usage, it is best to discuss this issue with your partner to guarantee you are both on the same page. See Chapter 14 - *How to Talk to Your Partner About Oral Sex* for some suggestions.

THE AMBIENCE

As already stated, preparing the pre-fellatio scene with a hot pumpkin pie and some liquorice spice may help to get your partner's juices flowing. Other more typical sensual scenes involve candles, music, finger food, low lighting, and easily removable or sexy clothing. That being said, in some cases, you can woo your partner by simply showing up naked. Consider your partner's likes, dislikes, turn-ons, and turn offs when setting the scene.

THE CLEAN UP

Towels, socks, facecloths, t-shirts, wet wipes, tissue, and hand cloths are all viable clean up aids if you don't plan on swallowing or if you simply have gotten lube and saliva everywhere. Keep these close by for easy clean up. You may also want to have a glass of water and some gum or breath mints nearby for a quick mouth wash and fresh mouth feel.

Aside from setting the scene with a little ambience and stocking up your bedside table with a few must-have, feel-good products, and safety paraphernalia, there isn't much else you need to worry about. The absence or presence of a cock piercing or foreskin may shock you, but you can always prepare yourself with an arsenal of blow job specific techniques aimed at pleasuring a penis with or without piercings and foreskin. See *Chapter 7 - Blow Job Positions* for ideas.

Doctors at the Smell and Taste Treatment and Research Centre hypothesize that pleasant odours—since they tend to positively increase other behaviours—would likely increase penile blood flow. Their data supported this hypothesis. However, they have noted that a multitude of mechanisms could be at play. The odours could induce a type of Pavlovian conditioned response, reminding partners of past or present sexual partners, or their favourite foods, thereby evoking nostalgic recall. Or the odours may simply be relaxing, or perhaps awaken the reticular activating system, making the men more alert to any sexual cues (resulting in an increase in penile blood flow). The odours may also act neurophysiologically (meaning affecting the physical and nervous system) as there is a direct pathway that connects the olfactory bulb to the septal nucleus, which induces blood flow and erection. Other possible explanations could exist, but the direct connection between odours and sexual response cannot be ignored or denied.

THE TEASE

Some people want to be ravished: a quick, passionate rip-your-clothes-off experience. Foreplay is minimal—and/or raw and aggressive—and getting down to the nitty-gritty is the name of the game. However, many great blow jobs require a little more time, and the art of a pleasurable tease. Just because your partner may be hard and ready to go, doesn't mean your mouth needs to invite them in, just yet.

TEASING 101

Here is a playful example of an artfully crafted how-to instructional guide to teasing ones male-bodied partner. This is by no means the only or right way to tease your mate, it is simply an example of how one individual may traverse these erotic waters.

Sara's Story

Before coming face to face with my partner's penis, I spend some time kissing and biting on his neck and ears, while at the same time whispering to him what's to come. I then unbutton his shirt and spend some time on his nipples (lick, flick, kiss, and blow). I make sure to hold myself back from taking all his clothes off at once though, undressing by layers feels far more seductive. I leave his underwear on while I kiss and nibble my way around his thighs and abs. I sometimes even bite his penis gently through his underwear and rub it softly with my hands through his clothes.

Once I start to feel my partner squirm, usually when I notice his hips push towards me, and I hear him telling me he's craving more...then and only then, do I allow my mouth to taste his penis. At this point he's usually begging for me to take his penis deep into my mouth, but I don't do it, at least not quite yet.

> *I slowly peel back his underwear, and then give a slow, long lick up his shaft and around the head. After this initial exploration I make direct eye contact and finally take his penis fully into my mouth. I take it all, and take it deep. If I'm feeling it, I moan to show my partner the pleasure I'm getting from this treat, a treat that only he can offer.*

This is the start of the dance called the tease, a dance not easily forgotten. Teasing doesn't only have to happen prior to commencing oral pleasure; rather it can also be a good way to prolong sensuality and can keep your partner begging for more.

That being said, teasing your partner every time you give oral sex may not be a good habit to get into. It may take away from the appeal and sensuality of the occasional tease, and could cause frustration in the most patient of individuals. You may want to use it instead as an intermittent or sporadic technique that you pull from your bag of tricks, not as an everyday go to.

"Lets flip a coin: heads I get tail, tails I get head"
– Unknown

7

Blow Job Positions

The Good, The Bad and The Upside-Down Inverted Flying Lotus

The Kama Sutra is often thought of as the most expansive literary work on sexual positioning. Some of its techniques and postures, however, could only be categorized as near impossible, and likely unpleasurable for either partner. Be that as it may, it is not our place to know what you are or are not capable of, and what you will or won't find stimulating. Therefore, we researched and compiled an extensive list of fellatio positions for your reading pleasure, as well as how to modify each position to suit your needs and pleasure buttons. While there was a great deal of work put into describing and modifying each of these, it would be pompous of us to claim that we 'invented' them and have the authority to name them. Therefore, allow us introduce you to the many names and faces of fellatio positioning.

POSITION #1

Also Known As: The Early Riser, Helping to Pitch the Tipi, Collecting Your Morning Wood

This is one of the most common positions. It involves your partner lying on their back with your head between their legs. As the giver, you are usually lying on your stomach, or resting on your knees. It's often called "The Early Riser" because many males are already in this position if/when they wake with a morning erection. It also doesn't require much movement, repositioning, or exuberance on either end; one simply needs to slip down a few feet and arouse your partner's package.

The Early Riser does give you good access to your partner's anus, penis and testicles (especially if they are willing to spread their legs so you can explore anal play); however, it doesn't provide your partner with a lot to look at. Most of your body is blocked from view, therefore using your sexy body as a visual aid or turn on for your partner—and/or playing with yourself occasionally while stimulating the penis—may be more difficult to do.

If your partner is a side sleeper you can still perform the Early Riser; simply slip down beneath the covers—while staying on your side— and give their package some morning love. This side positioning will allow them to thrust quite easily, and the mattress will provide you some much needed neck support. If your partner is feeling particularly frisky, flip yourself around and perform a lazy-man's 69, with both of you rested on your sides.

To bump this position up a notch, you may want to ask your partner to sit up slightly. Propping the head with a pillow, or using a headboard for support, can increase the visual component and give your partner a little something extra to look at. You could also try arching your back and sticking your beautiful behind in the air while performing "The Early Riser". The sway of your backside and the arch of your back is often found to add a touch more excitement to the visual scene. If your partner is game for anal play, have them spread their legs wide—or toss a foot or two up in the air—and you'll be good-to-go for below the belt access.

When switching between positions, you may find it helpful to maintain good eye contact. This can help keep the intimacy and sexual allure alive while you shift, fumble, and rearrange body parts.

POSITION #2

Also Known As: The Submissive Susie, Down On Bended Knee, Crouching Tiger Hidden Dragon, Praying for Some One-on-One Time

This position is often reported to be a favourite, due to its visuals and penile access. This position involves the giver kneeling down in front of their receiving partner. Many prefer to put a pillow under their knees for comfort, but depending on the location, this isn't always possible. This position gets its many names from the ever-so-obvious submissive pose, alluding to the fact that the receiver has the ultimate control and the giver is subservient to them. Although this is alluring to many from a fantasy standpoint, a few individuals in this kneeling position find that the subservient pose rubs them the wrong way. This is understandable, as the position does appear to place the giver in the obedient submissive role. However, appear is the key word here. Remember: you are always in control, you always have power, regardless of the position.

This position provides the receiver with great visuals, provides easy access, and plays into a common dominance fantasy. However, it can be uncomfortable for the giver and doesn't provide great anal access for those wanting to venture to the backdoor during oral sex.

To modify this position, allow the receiver to lean back up against a wall for support, or lean forward towards the wall with an outstretched arm to take some of the weight off their soon to be shaky knees. They can also position one leg up on a chair, evolving the "Submissive Susie" to "The Captain Morgan."

POSITION #3

Also Known As: The King's Throne, The Lazy Man's Holiday, The Ultimate Relaxation

This position is a lot like position #2 except instead of standing, your partner is sitting on a couch, chair, or any other horizontal surface. Some prefer this to "Submissive Susie" after they've had a long day or a hard workout, as it doesn't require them to use any real muscle strength. This can also be slightly more comfortable for the giver, as you are able to change positions, sit on your legs, and shift your body weight, all the while playing with your partner's penis and not missing a beat.

"The King's Throne" is considered to be quite popular because it is one of the most comfortable positions to both give and receive head. It can be quite relaxing for your partner—allowing them to fulfill their orgasm laden reclining La-Z-Boy® fantasies—and it doesn't do a number on your knees, back, or neck.

If you are in a living room scenario, you can throw a little more excitement into the mix by popping in an erotic movie (or any film that tickles your fancy). By providing that extra bit of audio and visual stimuli to the background, you may just kick your partner into full throttle and speed up the ejaculation process.

DID YOU KNOW?

Sex Pheromones were first identified in insects. These pheromones functioned as powerful come-hither signals, luring prospective mates from far away. Many nonhuman mammals also release sex-specific odorants. These are detected by a special sense organ in the nose called the VNO (vomeronasal organ). With the discovery of the VNO, science set out to uncover sexual pheromones in humans; however, what they found wasn't promising. After years of research, they determined that human sex pheromones may exist, but solid proof is hard to come by, and if they do, they are probably not sensed by the VNO—a relic of our evolutionary past—but rather our regular olfactory system. Factors such as where a female is in her menstrual cycle, and a male's testosterone level, may have more of an effect than the possible presence and detection of pheromones. Nonetheless, there are those who still believe that the olfactory system plays a central role in human sexuality (consciously perceived odours aside) perhaps even influencing traits such as sexual orientation.

POSITION #4

Also Known As: The Classy Lassie, The Dingo Down Under, The Weiner Dog

The "Classy Lassie" gets its name from its doggy style positioning. However, unlike the infamous intercourse arrangement, the giver is on all-fours facing the male's genitals (so your partner is in front of you receiving instead of behind you giving). This position is great for more aggressive deep throat action, as your partner can use your hips or butt as leverage to get a good pumping motion going; however, it does increase the probability of gagging.

The "Classy Lassie" provides your partner with great visuals, as they can see most of your body swaying back and forth as you work on expanding their pleasure. However, it's difficult to use both your hands as you will need one to support yourself during the process; therefore, you lose one crucial aid (the use of a pleasure providing appendage) throughout the entire experience. Nevertheless, many males report thoroughly enjoying this position and its raw, intercourse like motions.

To reduce the chances of gagging during quicker and deeper thrusting motions, simply remind your partner that your free hand will be placed gently around their testicles. If they thrust too deeply or start to get carried away, simply pull down slightly on the testicles. This will act as a 'slow down' warning and remind them to be more gentle.

If you prefer to be on two feet instead of on all fours (and yo taller bed frame/height), have your partner kneel on the edge of the bed. By standing on the floor and bending in half at your waist, you put your partner's penis directly in your eyesight, and you gain the use of both your hands.

You can also get your partner to stand on the edge of a bathtub, holding onto the curtain rail (assuming there is a solid place to stand). This can bring their penis closer to the level of your mouth —depending on your height ratios—so you don't have to bend over as much.

DID YOU KNOW?

Oral sex has become a far more common and widespread activity among our youth over the last few decades. Younger individuals are more likely than older individuals to have engaged in oral sex at some point during their lifetime. For example, in a British study, only approximately 50% of women and 62% of men within the 45-59 age bracket said that they had ever participated in any kind of oral sex; however, 83% of women and 88% of men in the 25-34 age bracket had done so. The famous Kinsey surveys of the 1940's reported much lower rates of oral sex than the present NHSLS and NSSAL surveys, suggesting that oral sex occurrence is in fact increasing as the years go by (or at least peoples willingness to admit to it).

POSTION #5

Also Known As: The 69, The Multitasker, The Numbers Game

The "69" is probably the most well-known oral sex position, deriving its name from the striking resemblance it bears to the actual number 69. Although it sounds good in theory, some find it to be a distracting position. If all of your focus and attention is directed towards what you are doing, not much mental energy may go towards actually receiving the pleasure you are given. Or you may zone out and take in all the pleasure, thereby giving poor oral sex in return.

The "69" doesn't provide good frontal visuals for you or your partner, however this position can provide you with a good deep throat angle (which is explained in more detail later in this chapter) and a close-up, eyeball full for those exploring anal play; however, the top bunk requires you to support yourself, adding fatigue and a decrease in hand playing availability.

Spin the "69" a mere 90 degrees by turning your body sideways so the two of you form the letter L instead of the number 69. This position gives your partner a great side view of your body and is perfect for those with a penis that is slightly curved to the left or right. If your partner leans to the left, saddle up to their left side. This may allow a curved penis to point down your throat with just the right angle.

You can also spin a slight 30 degrees—from the 69 position—to the left or right (so your knees and lower half are just over your partner's shoulder). This puts your privates just out of the range of their mouth, but close enough for them to use their hands to pleasure you, while watching you pleasure them. It is best if they are propped up slightly (with a pillow or headboard) so they can see the action happening, and so they have a better reach in order to hit your more intimate areas.

POSITION #6

Also Known As: The Upside-Down Flying Superman, The Mechanic, Deep Throat Done Right

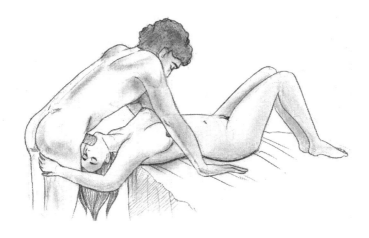

The "Upside-Down Flying Superman" is not a highly practiced and well-known position, which is unfortunate, as it's renowned for its ease into the deep throating world. Position yourself on your back laying across the bed, so that your head and neck hang over the side of the mattress. Your partner then stands on the ground and squats just slightly (depending on the height of your bed), positioning themselves facing you so that they can enter your mouth with ease. The angle of your neck allows the penis to slide down your throat effortlessly, and your gag reflex can take a much needed hiatus.

The "Upside-Down Flying Superman" can sometimes cause the odd head rush. Be that as it may, it is still an amazing position for your partner's visual stimuli as your whole body is on display and it can be really helpful for those who struggle with a sensitive gag reflex. It is also an excellent pose for more aggressive oral sex, allowing your partner to thrust into your mouth with a vigour that closely resembles penetrative intercourse.

Many individuals find that they simply can't keep their hands to themselves when viewing an outstretched body sprawled out before them. Therefore, the positive side of the head rush coin is that your partner is in the perfect position to use both of their hands to play with your body. Depending on the height differential, they should be able to reach any and all erotic areas that you allow them to venture into.

POSITION #7

Also Known As: The Tanned Banana Peeler, Big Breasted Blowing Beauty, Bringing in the Ladies

In order to perform The "Tanned Banana Peeler" correctly, you must have breasts. Now this isn't to say that men can't participate, as they have their own version—a.k.a. "The Lazy Larry"—however, to really perfect the position, breasts work best. Start out by lying on your back. A bed, couch, or any flat surface will work, but having an object to prop your head up with is crucial. Then simply push your breasts together so that you create a well-formed space between them for the penis to slide. Every time your partner thrusts between your breasts and their penis peaks out between them, aim to give it some good oral loving.

This position is great for large breasted women, or those who find it difficult, uncomfortable, or are just uninterested in deep throating (as your breasts take the majority of the penis length, allowing only part of your partner's penis to enter your mouth). Many love the visual combination of your chest with your mouth; however, with both your hands occupied, it doesn't allow for much variation in technique, and your accessibility is quite limited.

To help your partner's penis glide, you may want to add some edible lubrication to your breasts. Some chocolate and banana flavoured lubricant may entice you to lick away, and your partner will feel a warmer more natural glide. If you have smaller breasts—or you've got some lovely nipples but no breasts at all—don't get discouraged. Use your hands and fingers to increase your breast tunnel length (or the amount of surface area their penis comes into contact with before reaching your mouth) near the top of your chest. By using your hands as a tunnel, with the mouth as the end point, you will provide your partner with all the stimulation they need, regardless of whether you've got large breasts, or a flat muscular chest.

POSITION #8

Also Known As: Top Dog, The Personal Trainer, Pumping Push-up

The "Top Dog" is a lot like the well-known missionary position; however, instead of looking into each other's eyes, you slide down under the covers and face the penis. Your partner remains on top, in the missionary or push-up position, and you remain on your back, but half way down the bed, facing your partners genitals.

If you aren't prone to gagging, this is a good lazy way to give head. One simply slides down a few feet and lets their partner do all the work. In this position, your partner can thrust in a sex-like fashion and you simply get to lie there and wait for the finale. However, if this thrusting technique doesn't appeal to you, and/ or your partner would like a few more visuals during oral sex, then the "Top Dog" is probably not for you. This position does allow for two free hands to explore anal or ball play, but one's eyesight—to traverse through and discover these areas—is extremely limited.

To help control the speed of thrusting, place your hands on their butt and hips and guide then with gentle pushing, pulling, or squeezing. By placing one hand on the front of their upper thigh, in their groin area beside their penis, you can also control the depth they are allowed to enter.

You can adjust this position by having your partner lay on their side instead of in the push-up position above you. You would lay on your back with your head tilted sideways towards your partner's penis. In this position they are still able to thrust towards you while on their side and you are able to use your hands to pleasure yourself. This creates a great visual for your partner (as they watch you pleasuring yourself) and it creates the opportunity for you to orgasm together.

POSITION #9

Also Known As: Sleepy Susie, Lazy Lounger, Breakfast of Champions

The "Sleepy Susie" gets its name from the fact that you are giving oral sex in the position that many people wake up in—lying flat on your back with a pillow under your head. Your partner does most of the work by positioning themselves on their knees straddling your face.

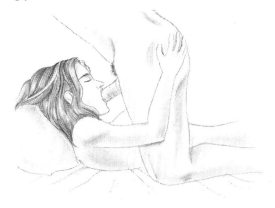

This position is great for times when the giver just wants to sit back and enjoy the ride. Many males enjoy face thrusting in this position as the giver is not able to do many head movements (back and forth, up and down) as their head is resting on the pillow. This doesn't mean that the giver shouldn't still use their hands to please their partner, but head movements are generally kept to a minimum. Although this position is a great lazy man's option to giving head, the anal visuals are minimal.

Use one hand to stimulate your partner's penis and your other hand to stimulate yourself. The "Sleepy Susie" is a great position for mutual orgasms/pleasure as you can use your free hand to stimulate yourself while your partner enjoys their penis thrusting mouth play.

POSITION #10

Also Known As: Inverted Flying Lotus, The Stand-Worthy 69, The He-Man, Standing Room Only

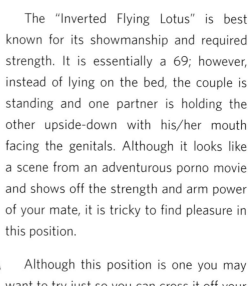

The "Inverted Flying Lotus" is best known for its showmanship and required strength. It is essentially a 69; however, instead of lying on the bed, the couple is standing and one partner is holding the other upside-down with his/her mouth facing the genitals. Although it looks like a scene from an adventurous porno movie and shows off the strength and arm power of your mate, it is tricky to find pleasure in this position.

Although this position is one you may want to try just so you can cross it off your list of experimentations, we have yet to meet a couple who enjoy this as a regular go-to for mutual pleasure or orgasm achievement. The upside down partner often complains of head rushes and the inability to get a real speed or rhythm going with regards to their 'performance,' and the standing partner often complains about the strength it takes to hold a person for long enough in that position to obtain any real long-term pleasure.

This position also requires a minimum height differential, as it's nearly impossibly to do a standing 69 if there is a drastic difference in the length of the torsos.

If your partner is able to lean against a wall, preferably a slanted wall, it will help ease some of the weight they must hold. Alternatively, they can also sit (or rest their butt slightly) on the edge of the arm of a couch or high bed/mattress.

8

Tips and Techniques

The How To, Must Not's and the "Seriously People Do That?!" Section

1. DEPLOYING EXTRA TROOPS

As stated in the new definition of oral sex in chapter one, it takes a lot more than the use of one's mouth to perform fellatio. Using your hand, or hands, to simulate the feeling of deep penetration can be an important part of giving head. Think of your hand as an extension of your mouth, moving in tandem. As you bob your head up and down on your partner's shaft, your mouth is focused on the head—where the skin is most sensitive —and your hand on the base of the penis, where it is the least sensitive. When they move together, they create the illusion of a long deeply penetrating orifice. Using these extra appendages as pleasure givers also provides your mouth with the occasional R&R time, and it allows you to try out a good number of the other techniques listed below. You can also up the intimacy factor by reaching out and holding hands with your partner during oral sex (if you have a hand to spare) or put a finger in their mouth for them to lick or suck on while you pleasure the troops down below.

See the *Handy Man's Corner* in the *Advanced Techniques* section for a stylistic how-to on using your hands during oral sex.

DID YOU KNOW?

An article was written on the hazards of oral sex—by a group of dentists—and published in a medical journal (Bellizi, Krakow and Plack, Military Medicine 145 (1980):787 – Yes the dentists name is really Dr. Plack...you can't make this stuff up). The article speaks of one unfortunate soul, the daughter of a soldier who was taken to the base hospital because she discovered a discoloration in the back of her mouth. After much research and debate the dentists finally discovered the cause of the black-and-blue blotch near her tonsils. Proceeding very diplomatically, the doctors asked the father to leave the room while they posed a very delicate question to the young girl: "Do you have a boyfriend?" Near where the tonsils hang is a highly vascularised mass of tissues. An erect penis hitting up against this sensitive tissue—as the dentists discovered— can therefore cause bruising. The bruise, like any other, will go away in time however, it is a gentle reminder to take it easy on your partner's oral cavity, as no one wants to have to explain that medical diagnosis to anyone.

2. FOCUSING ON THE FRENULUM

The Frenulum is located on the underside of the penis in the subtle V-shaped site that circles around the head of the penis. This is often known as the most sensitive part; therefore focusing

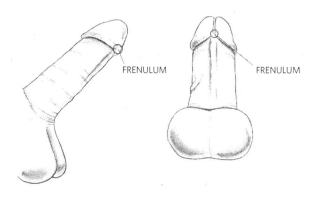

FRENULUM   FRENULUM

some titillating tongue time on this area can do wonders to heighten pleasure. Just be careful not to give too much direct attention—or too much pressure—to this treasure spot, as there is a very fine line between pleasure and pain.

3. TITILLATING TONGUE TIME: TONGUE-TWISTERS FOR THE BJ SAVVY

Tip #1 Fat tongue vs. Skinny tongue

Some people enjoy a lollipop lick. This action is just as it sounds, a wide tongue to cover more surface area and a slow lick up the shaft taking in as much of the lollipop as you can. Remember that there is a "seam" on a male's privates that runs from just below the head to halfway down the scrotum; if you are feeling adventurous you can venture beneath the testes to the perineum or anus. Other people prefer a more localized licking; this involves a skinny or pointed tongue that focuses on one specific area of the penis (such as the corona or frenulum). A combo gives you the best chance of hitting the sweet spot.

Tip #2 The Flicker vs. The Tornado

As the name implies, the flicker is a quick tongue movement that is akin to those made by a very thirsty animal. It is best used on sensitive areas—such as the frenulum—and done in brief interludes. The Tornado is a circular motion that can be done on its own (your tongue outside your mouth focusing on going around the head of the penis) or in combination with the typical up-and-down strokes done with your mouth and hand (tongue stays inside your mouth). If you're doing the Tornado while keeping your tongue inside your mouth, keep it positioned normally (as if you were sucking your thumb) for the down stroke on the penis; however, on the way up pause ever so slightly to do a quick once around with your tongue on the head of the penis, without breaking oral contact, and then continue back down the shaft. Repeat.

Tip #3 The Strap On vs. The Cubby Hole

The tongue can be a very useful aid in providing vibrations through the use of mini/bullet vibrators that fit in the mouth. These are pill sized vibrators that can sit underneath your

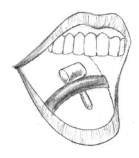

tongue or slide onto your tongue. The Strap On is a vibrator that is attached to a small stretchy band that fits around your tongue; you can position this just right so that any penis-tongue touching done with the tip of your tongue will produce extra sensations.

The Cubby Hole works in much the same way except you place the bullet in that small space under your tongue where is stays put with no band to hold it in place; this allows you to do up and down strokes without the vibrator "harness" being felt by the receiver, and it opens up the opportunity to give the testes some tickling sensations. Some people love the Cubby Hole technique when you engulf a testicle in your mouth while using your free hands to play and explore.

4. TAKE TIME FOR THE TESTES

It's easy to get carried away with your partner's penis and forget that they have other parts that could use some attention as well. Massaging the testicles—and the area in between—can be quite pleasurable (just don't get too carried away as they aren't stress balls). Some people enjoy this massaging motion of the testicles while your mouth focuses on the shaft; however, don't forget to occasionally take each testicle into your mouth and hum or suck on it, as that can be a pleasurable add-on to your typical penis-to-mouth show.

There are many ways to caress the testicles; here are a few that rate well:

Position your thumb in between the two testicles. With a generous amount of lubricant slide your finger up and down between the two balls applying enough pressure to massage the base of the penis.

Pull the loose skin from around the testis to either side of the balls and then massage that skin between your fingertips (think of it like pulling your skin away from your elbow and then rubbing that loose skin back and forth).

Rest the palm of your hand over your partner's penis with your fingertips pointed down towards their anus. Lightly massage the back part of the scrotum (where it attaches to the body) and caress their balls with your fingers. While your fingers move, so will the part of your wrist that's resting on their penis. This provides subtle penis pleasure while your fingertips explore their testicles.

5. GAG PREVENTION

It's pretty rare to find an individual who likes gagging. Therefore, to minimize the chances of choking on your partner's package, consider these five tips:

Tip #1 Bringing in the Big Guns

By placing one hand at the base of your partners penis you automatically gain four knuckles worth of buffer space, leaving no more than a few inches to enter your mouth (if your partner is of average length). If your partner is well endowed, simply use two hands—like you're holding a bat—instead of one.

Tip #2 Positioning

To stop your partner from involuntary thrusting when they are about to cum, keep them on their back. Position yourself in between their legs and rest your forearms and a portion of your body weight on your partner's upper thighs and pelvis. The weight of your body will help discourage any upwards thrusting. If they still have the desire and power to thrust towards your face, your whole body will come up with them.

DID YOU KNOW?

Although the withdrawal (withdrawal method/"pull-out" method) can be highly effective, with perfect use ranging at about 96% effective, the rate for typical use of this method is closer to 73% successful. This means that in general 27/100 individuals using this method of intercourse will get pregnant. This is because pre-cum can contain semen, and some males aren't quick enough to always withdraw the penis before some semen has been released.

Tip #3 Grab the Reins to Control the Bucking Bronco

Place one hand gently around their scrotum (with your thumb and forefinger around the upper section, where the testicles attach to the groin). With your partner's testicles in the palm of your hand, lightly pull downwards if/when they start to thrust. The more they thrust, the more you increase your downward pull. Some people find this pleasurable, others you'll have to scrape off the roof if you tug too aggressively. Be gentle, but remember that you are in control and to pull those reins if your partner gets a little too forceful and excited.

Tip #4 Be Vocal

Yes, this can be tough to do with a penis in your mouth, but timing is everything. It is important to speak up for what you like, don't like, and what is acceptable in the bedroom. If you are gagging and don't like it, you need to tell your partner. Explain the difference between good facial thrusting and bad (if you feel there is a difference) and help them learn. Don't let anyone gag you or thrust too aggressively if it hurts or is outside your comfort zone.

Tip #5 Refer to Blow Job Position #6 "Deep Throat Done Right"

This position allows for deep throat penetration while minimizing the chances of the uncontrollable gag reflex. It provides the perfect angle for insertion and is high on the visual stimulation index, as your whole body is on display.

6. THE SOUNDS OF PLEASURE: A REAL HUMDINGER

A blow job is not just about using your mouth as an entry point, it's also about using it for verbal communication. You may want to moan with delight, or occasional throw out words of encouragement, to boost your partner's confidence. If you need help mustering up some sexy honesty, cover your partner's penis in flavoured lubricant, wait until they have fully risen to the occasion, and focus on parts of their body that you do find attractive. You may also want to use your sounds of pleasure to hum while engulfing the penis in your mouth. Some people love a good humdinger while their head and frenulum are in your mouth. If you're struggling with ideas for what to sing, hum the alphabet and find out what your partner's favourite letters are!

"Graze on my lips; and if those hills be dry, stray lower, where the pleasant fountains lie."
– William Shakespeare

7. KING KONG

When giving oral sex to a partner who is well endowed it may be helpful to use two hands on the shaft and/or pump the shaft while focusing your oral efforts on just the frenulum and head. You can also try a sideways oral massage by laying the penis against your partners stomach so it's pointing towards their head, then use one hand to caress their testicles and the other hand to cradle/squeeze their penis (so your hand is between the penis and the abdomen area, resting on the stomach). Use a lot of saliva and plenty of tongue to "french kiss" this frenulum area while stroking your partner's shaft. Every so often fill your hands with your hot steamy breath and extra saliva. This is also an effective technique in getting your partner to cum orally without swallowing.

8. LIPS IN DISGUISE

Drawing attention to the lips can increase visual stimulation. The mouth and lips serve as an evolutionary billboard for arousal because the more sexually turned on you get, the more blood flows to your face, and mouth, as well as those delicate areas between a female's legs. Increased blood flow therefore, makes things larger and redder then they would normally appear. The more turned on your partner thinks you are (by observing these visuals), the more turned on they become. In short, lips can be a visible vulva; no wonder red lipstick has been the most popular colour throughout the ages!

Anything that you can do to draw attention to your mouth is considered prolonged foreplay. Many claim that one of their biggest turn-ons is watching their partner eat an ice cream cone. You can imagine the direct correlation between hands wrapped around the cone, and one's tongue working feverishly to catch all the drips with a look of glee upon getting your favourite treat. The same rules apply for lollipops or any finger foods. Screw the napkins; tactfully licking or sucking the last morsels off of your fingers will plant a thought that can get their mind racing.

The largest sexual organ in humans is our brains, therefore laying the ground work throughout the day can make even an everyday blow job seem like the best they've ever had. Whether that means spending a little extra time on that ice cream cone, or sexting your partner about what's to "cum", you can't go wrong with a little extra tease.

9. TO CUM WITHOUT WARNING

Most people know when they reach the point of no return and are about to ejaculate, so if you don't want your partner to ejaculate in your mouth, just say so. Ask them to tell you when they're about to cum so you can pull your mouth away; after a while you will probably start to learn your partner's signs and will no longer need the heads up.

Possible signs your partner may be ready to fire:

- The penis starts to swell a little larger and may contort slightly.
- The testicles draw closer to their body.
- Their abs or ass tighten and their hips give a forward thrust.
- Their legs straighten, their head tilts back, their hands make a fist, and their toes begin to stretch or curl.
- They begin screaming: "Oh God, I'm cumming!"

Swallowing is a personal preference and your comfort level in doing so may change over time and between partners. To swallow or not so swallow is your decision therefore the "heads up" should always be given by your partner unless you state otherwise; it is simply common courtesy. If you aren't comfortable swallowing, or having any kind of oral semen intake, simply wait for their cue—or watch for the signs of ejaculation —and then free your mouth from the line of fire, however don't stop stimulating them. Slide your hand up the shaft, just below the head, and start feverishly pumping the shaft. Make sure you have a firm grip while you pump quickly (with a well-lubricated hand). Don't stop these quick pumping motions until the last few drops of ejaculate have been dispensed.

10. THE TASTE OF SUCCESS

If the taste of your partner's semen is something you just can't stomach, try this technique for reducing taste-bud-to-semen contact. When it feels like your partner is close to coming (or they have given you the heads up that they are ready to fire) place your tongue over the head of their penis. The first shot will hit the underside of your tongue where there aren't any taste buds. The ejaculate will then ooze down their shaft or flow quickly from your mouth and away from your taste buds. Another trick is to start mobilizing a pool of saliva in your mouth when you feel they are getting close to erupting. When they cum let the floodgates of slobber loose. The saliva will help to thin out the ejaculate and cause it to run out of your mouth at a quicker pace. On the flip side, you could also roll a condom over your partner's penis reducing the possibility of getting any ejaculate in your mouth (See the *Advanced Techniques* Chapter for a how-to guide).

If you're looking for other effective ways to mask the taste of semen, check out Chapter 10 - *Who Said You Shouldn't Play With Your Food.*

DID YOU KNOW?

Female fruit bats have been shown to lower their heads during intercourse in order to run their tongues along the shaft or base of the penis. A positive relationship has been shown to exist between the length of time the female licked the penis and the duration of copulation time (having sex), meaning that mating pairs have been shown to spend significantly more time in copulation if this type of oral sex was preformed, then if the activity was absent. But don't worry ladies, the female bat doesn't go uncompensated. The males also show post-copulatory genital grooming after intercourse—an important quality for any sexually intelligent species.

9

Advanced Techniques

Neapolitan:

A term used to define sex (or foreplay) that is varied, kinky, imaginative, exotic, interesting, or exciting. In this chapter you will need to explore your Neapolitan side. Some of these techniques you and/or your partner may love or hate, and others may cause sudden and unexpected bursts of ejaculatory pleasure—you be the judge.

11. VIBRATORS - NOT JUST FOR SOLO FUN.

You can use either a bullet or dildo shaped tool to trace their penis, tickle their balls, venture out to their nipples, or explore their undercarriage; the places are virtually endless. If done correctly, a tactfully placed vibrator can send your partner into another dimension. You can also hold a vibrator against the outside of your cheek or against your jaw bone to allow the vibrations to spread through your mouth to their member. Think of it like humming, only on steroids. Also, check out the previous Chapter for the description on tongue vibrators.

If your partner is open to the idea of back door pleasure, you can also try inserting a small vibrator up their anus. Some people claim that the most intense orgasms they have ever had have come from the combination of a blow job and a vibrating object pushing up against their prostate. Just make sure that you are using a vibrator that is designed for anal play, as the anus tends to suck things up inside and then refuses to return them.

A word to the wise: if you are going to be using vibrators or toys with your partner make sure that you are cleaning and sterilizing them between each use (as you should be even if they

DID YOU KNOW?

You may be surprised to know that not all semen are swimmers with a one-track mind of egg fertilization, there are actually three different types of semen. One type of sperm are the "hunters," their only job is to seek out and destroy or immobilize sperm from any other male. The second type of sperm are the "blockers," their job is to form a barrier or wall so that other sperm coming after them are unable to get by and reach the eggs. The third type of sperm are the most well-known as they are the "fertilizers," they seek out the egg and make a connection. All three work together in order to give the "fertilizers" the best chance at success.

are just for personal use). Also, a vibrator that has been used in the anus should never be inserted into the vagina unless it has been properly sterilized first, due to potential bacterial and viral transfer.

"I like to see oral sex, manual sex and intercourse as foreplay for my vibrator sex." – Betty Dodson

12. COCK SLEEVE – A LAZY LOVER'S BEST FRIEND

A cock sleeve can be a fun aid to boost pleasure but must be used carefully, as in some cases it can work so well that your

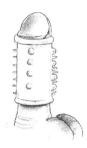

partner may have trouble lasting longer than a few seconds before ejaculating. To use, simply add a few drops of lube to the inside of the silicone tube and then slide it over the shaft of the penis. There are different varieties—some with only one opening—so look for a cock sleeve that has two holes. Once the sleeve is in place, gently stroke the sleeve up and down as you place your mouth over the head of the penis.

13. COCK RING

The cock ring can be used for many different purposes, such as helping your partner to cum faster and/or for holding the blood within their penis if they have trouble maintaining erections. Cock rings come in a variety of shapes, sizes and textures. Some have vibrating bullets, others are metal, but most are silicone rings that look like rubber bands. If your partner has trouble maintaining an erection during sex or foreplay simply place a silicone cock ring down at the base of their penis. Cock rings are meant to be tight (as its job is to hold the blood in the shaft) so you shouldn't be able to slide the ring down—like you would a condom—but rather you must stretch it and place it in position. Some individuals prefer to place the cock ring around the base of their penis and around their testicles, others find more pleasure and function just placing it at the base of the penis shaft. Both versions are fine and can be pleasurable however if the main goal is to aid in the retention of the erection (keeping a firm erection) then not including the testicles in this cock ring placement is a more effective technique. If you just want to give your partner a little extra stimulation, purchase a vibrating cock ring. This will hold the vibrator in place at the base of their penis while you use your free hands to give pleasure and explore.

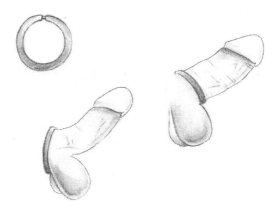

14. COLD CAN BE HOT

Keep a glass of ice cubes or crushed ice nearby to allow for a variety of temperature teasing possibilities. The most straightforward involves you allowing a small amount of ice to melt in your mouth, or holding a bit of the cold water in your mouth for a moment prior to wrapping your lips around the head of your partner's penis. The cold will last for a short time, while offering a new sensation for your partner to discover. You can also dribble the cold water over their penis (in this case, less is more). Likewise, you can try placing the ice cube in your mouth and allowing it to melt as you shower your partners penis with love. However, be mindful not to leave the ice cube on any one spot for too long as it can go from pleasure to pain faster than you think. Alternatively, you can hold the ice cube in your hand and switch between using your mouth and running the ice cube along the shaft or allowing it to drip down the shaft as it melts in your hand.

Beyond the H2O

If you're not a fan of the ice cubes try putting grapes in the freezer and popping a few of those in your mouth. You can drive them wild by rolling the grapes around their penis with your tongue, or filling each side of your cheeks with grapes (frozen or thawed) as you go up and down their shaft. A word to the wise, this could also be a choking hazard, so play with care. If you have a tongue piercing, try placing the bar bell in the fridge or freezer before giving your partner head. This offers both hot and cold sensations from the same organ: your illustrious tongue.

DID YOU KNOW?

"Snowballing" is the name given to the act of allowing ejaculate to enter your mouth and then holding it there for a few brief moments while you make your way from your partners groin, to their mouth. A kiss is then exchanged between you and your partner so that the ejaculate can be transferred to their mouth, essentially giving them back their semen to swallow, gargle, and enjoy (if they're into that). Yes this is a real thing and no, not all people enjoy this. It is strongly advised that you check with your partner before catching them off-guard with a mouthful of their best swimmers.

15. SOME LIKE IT HOT

As with cold sensations, the feeling of warmth can awaken the pleasure senses. By holding some hot liquid in your mouth —such as tea or hot water—you are adding new sensations that are stronger, and warmer, than what your mouth can provide. Peppermint tea or a few powerful mints may also add a little tingle, just be careful that the liquid isn't too warm as burning your partner's penis isn't good for anyone. Some also report using warm water and "popping candy," however the reviews are still out as to whether that tickles, is painful, or a sensation overload of good times.

Playing with sensations: Once your partners penis is in your mouth (as far down as you can go or deep throating) start breathing in, then while taking air into your lungs move back up the shaft so you finish at the head of their penis with lungs full of air. Then let the air out slowly as you travel back down the penis resulting in a cool upstroke and a warm down stroke.

16. SCARVES

Purchase yourself a lovely silk scarf (or another soft and smooth material). A long and skinny one is ideal, but any one will do. For a bit of fun foreplay, wrap the scarf lightly around the shaft of the penis a few times, then gently and slowly pull on one end of the scarf so it slides around and off the penis. Make sure not to pull too quickly or it may tighten and be unpleasant.

For another way to make the scarf an accessory your partner won't soon forget, place the center of the scarf under their testicles and tie the ends snugly around and above the shaft. Hold the two scarf ends in one hand and place their penis in your mouth. Gently tug upwards on the scarf ends in time with your mouth strokes heading down their penis. This creates a pulsing sensation. Be mindful not to pull too hard or tie the scarf too tightly. Also you may want to choose a scarf you actually like and find fashionable as an added bonus. Each time you wear it out on the town, you are planting the seed about what's to come, driving your partner wild with anticipation, and filling their mind with past sexual memories. Let the tease begin. Scarves also make a great blindfold that can leave your lovers other senses heightened, making those sucking and caressing motions that much more intense and pleasurable.

17. PEARLS – THE GIFT THAT KEEPS GIVING

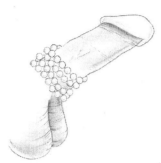

Now unfortunately this technique calls for the real thing. If you try this go-to-penis-pleaser with imitation pearls or other man-made beads, the seam edge may catch on the penis and cause a painful and very un-sexy situation. Nature simply knows how to do it best.

To begin add a few drops of lubricant to the shaft and then wrap the pearl necklace around the penis until it forms a coil up the shaft. Then gently roll the necklace up and down the penis. You can also use your mouth to add extra stimulation to the head of the penis, as the pearls roll up and down in pleasurable synchronicity. Just like the scarf technique—if you enjoying wearing necklaces—these pearls add a few extra hours of visual foreplay during dinner. You may want to take the time to play with the necklace throughout the night, rolling it through your fingertips as you talk.

18. PREPARING FOR A HAIR-RAISING ADVENTURE

If you have long locks why not put them to use? If your partner is lying down and your jaw needs a little break you can keep the energy flowing by running your hair over their chest, penis, and inner thighs. This can give a similar effect or feeling as using a feather, just be mindful of their body language as they could be ticklish. If you have really long locks to work with you can use a technique similar to that with the scarf. Slowly wrap a section of your hair under the scrotum and hold the end with your free hand, then tug up slightly as your head rises and release slightly as your head goes back down.

19. GIVING THE GOALIE SOME FACE TIME: PUTTING ON A CONDOM WITH YOUR MOUTH

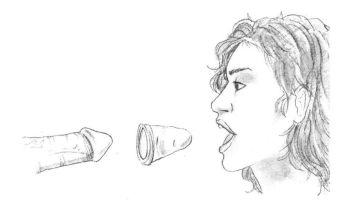

Although some people are not a fan of condoms, they are a first line, preventative measure that makes sex in all forms less risky—this includes oral sex (See the Risks/Safety Precautions section for more on this topic). So for the purposes of this book, it is assumed that unless you are with a committed partner or partners in a trusting relationship, condoms are being used. That being said, there are ways to make donning the condom more fun for everyone.

Step 1: Open the condom package. You can do this with your hands or your mouth.

If you wear lipstick, this would be the time to highlight your oral visual vulva with some deep red lipstick.

Step 2: Remove the condom from the wrapper and determine which way is the right side up (i.e. if you were to hold the tip of the condom between your fingers, you would be able to roll the condom downwards.

Placing a drop or two of lube on the inside of the tip of the condom will allow for more movement and glide and create a more natural lubricated feel for your partner. Try experimenting with cooling, tingling, or heating lubricants to add another dimension or sensation to the BJ experience, just be careful to not use too much as the condom may slip off.

Step 3: Using your open lips and some slight suction (imagine drinking from a straw), place the tip of the condom (the side you would hold to roll it down) in your mouth. Do not use your teeth as this can compromise the condom and impact its effectiveness.

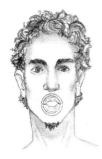

Step 4: While holding the condom partially in your mouth and against your lips, position your mouth above the head of the penis; let the penis gradually enter your mouth. By keeping your lips firm, the condom will slowly begin to work its way down the shaft.

If you need a little help making sure the condom is properly in position, bring in your hands to help guide the condom down to the base of the shaft while still using your mouth.

Step 5: Once you've got the condom completely unrolled and positioned onto the penis, use your hand to secure it in place at the base of the shaft as you work your way back up, and down, up and down, up and down...you get the picture.

20. CLEARING OUT THE PIPES

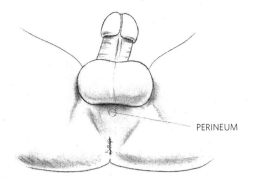

PERINEUM

After your partner ejaculates they may feel the urge to use their fingers to reach down and push out any cum that may still be in the pipes. How can they do this you ask? By massaging and gently pushing on their perineum (the area between the testicles and the anus). Now not all individuals do this, but for some it's the final finish—like giving the penis a couple good shakes after a pee. However, it's suggested you run this play by your partner before giving it a try as they may be baffled by your post cum care if they never thought to give it a go.

21. BALL TRICK

While using your hand to stroke your partner's penis in a fluid, rapid up-and-down motion, you may want to push your little finger—of your stroking hand—against the lower part of the shaft near their scrotum. This finger placement causes the testicles to jiggle or vibrate with each stroke. Some people love the added sensation however beware of your pinky nail length, as stabbing their balls with each up-and-down motion is bound to get an unpleasant reaction.

Fun times with the testes: Bobbing for Balls—get your partner to use their PC muscles (Pubococcygeus muscles) to move their penis up and down while you are on your knees (with your hands behind your back), bobbing for their penis and balls like a moving target. If your partner isn't sure where or what to "squeeze," the best way to locate the PC muscles is ask your partner to stop the flow of urine the next time they go to the washroom. The muscles they squeeze to stop the flow of urine are the PC muscles; these are what they would contract during your bobbing for balls fun.

22. SEXY PLEASURE WITH PRESSURE

While working your way downtown slowly, spend some time kissing your partners neck, ears, and nipples. Then reach down between their legs and start stroking their penis. While facing them, place your thigh in between their legs so it is gently pushing up against their testicle area. Be careful not to pinch their balls, as this is not meant to trap or squash their groin, but to add some stimulation and pressure to the root of their penis (perineum area) while giving them a pre-stroke tease before your mouth reaches its final destination.

23. HANDY MAN'S CORNER

Giving head involves the use of your hands; giving great head involves employing actual hand techniques. Here in the Handy Man's Corner, you get the run-down of how to use those appendages with style to create a blow job experience that's different every time.

Fists in Fluid Motion

Making sure the penis is generously lubed, wrap one hand around the base of the penis—and while squeezing lightly—pull it all the way up the shaft and up into the air. This party is not just for one hand however, you need to keep both hands flowing in the same upward motion from the base of the shaft up into the air, one hand right after the other. Make sure one hand is always at the base of the penis just as the other has left the head. Some folks also like to give a little extra squeeze on the upward stroke just as your hand reaches the head of the penis. You can also do this hand technique by moving your hands in the opposite direction (from the head to the base of the penis) however this requires a ready to go erection and a more open grip.

Praying for a Release

This is perfect for the "Kings Throne Blow Job Position" (See Chapter 7 - *Blow Job Positions*) as you want to place yourself directly in front of your partner's groin (kneeling so you are at eye level with it would be best). Interlock your fingers together as if you were in a deep prayer. Then use the inside pads of your hands to stroke your partners penis up and down—thumbs should be pointing upwards. Good technique as a starter to get them warmed up or as an interlude between penis-to-mouth action.

Bottle Cap Twist Off

Just like the name implies this action is akin to twisting off the cap of a bottle. With one hand hold the base or shaft of the penis and with your other hand grasp the head of the penis. Making sure your partner's penis is well lubricated, twist your hand around the head of the penis as though you were going to twist the top off of a bottle. This action requires a gentle motion with your thumb and forefinger running along the groove under the ridge (corona) where the head meets the shaft.

Wringing out the Towel

Place a generous amount of lube on the penis and then grasp the lower part of the shaft with one hand. Place the other hand on the upper part of the shaft being mindful not to leave a gap between your two hands. Then gently twist your hands back and forth in opposite directions as if you were wringing a towel dry. If your partner is well endowed, or you have small hands, be careful that you don't pinch the penis skin between your hands.

The Siskel and Ebert

Turn your hand upside-down—as if you were giving someone a 'thumbs down'—and then place that well-lubricated hand over the penis with your thumb at the base of the shaft. Bring the hand upwards (allowing your thumb to pass directly over the frenulum) until the tip of your thumb has reached the tip or head of the penis. Then roll the palm of your hand over the head as you flip to a thumbs up position. Move back downward towards the base of the penis. Repeat in reverse. Use your free hand to cup the balls and give a gentle massage or lightly tug down on them.

The Parachute

Place the palm of your hand over the top of the penis and let your fingers drop down along the sides of the shaft. This hand formation is akin to that of a parachute or octopus. Then use your fingers to stimulate, tickle, caress, and stroke the corona and shaft. You can also twist your hand sideways—embodying the corkscrew technique—and move your hand up and down so your fingers stimulate the sides of your partner's penis.

Perineum Massage

Many people assume that the penis embodies only what you can see. That it is somehow popped on to the pelvic bone and only the parts that show are the parts that matter. However, in reality the penis runs beneath the testicles. Some people find that massaging this "invisible" part of the penis, all the way back to where the anus begins, can be extremely pleasurable. There is an area on this part of the penis where a number of muscle fibers, nerve endings, and ligaments converge. Using fingertip pressure and massaging motions on this perineal area while you are giving oral sex can shoot some people into ecstasy.

24. PROSTATE PLEASURE

Although this book is not a "how-to" on anal sex, we couldn't write an all-inclusive book on blow jobs without including a little prostate play. You can find the prostate by sticking your finger about two inches up into the rectum (See Anatomy Chapter). You should make sure your fingernails are well trimmed, the anus —and your finger(s)—are well lubricated, and you ideally have a finger condom handy. Start by massaging the anus or entrance gently before diving right into finger insertion. Then slowly push your finger in a couple inches and start exploring. If your partner is lying on their back, you may want to make a slight "come here" motion (curling your fingers up towards their bellybutton). The texture of the prostate should resemble the feeling of the tip of your nose or the padded part of your thumb where it meets your wrist. Now stimulating the prostate alone will most likely not make your partner ejaculate, therefore it generally would need to be done in conjunction with some Handy Man's Corner techniques, and/or oral sex. When your partner is getting close to the "point of no return" (they are about to ejaculate) their prostate might feel like it's starting to dome or swell. At this moment it would be a good idea to gently push down on, or rub your finger around, the prostate. Applying finger pressure while your partner is cumming results in an ejaculation most refer to as a "gusher." If you are already a little queasy when it comes to ejaculate, then you may want to remove your mouth from your partner's penis for this orgasm explosion. As always, discuss your partner's comfort level with this before attempting.

25. THE TURTLE COVER & FORESKIN FUN

Many individuals don't get to choose if they keep their foreskin or not, as it's most often decided for them soon after birth by a parent or guardian. Those who do make it to adulthood with an intact foreskin have been compared to their hoodless counterparts in many ways. For example, research shows that penises with foreskins tend to be slightly more sensitive than penises without, however, every individual is different and many factors can

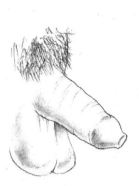 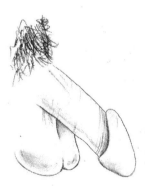

contribute to a person's level of sensitivity and arousal. Typically, most foreskins pull back when a male becomes erect, almost disappearing from view as they hug the base of the penis. This makes giving head to any person, once they are aroused, generally the same across the board. That being said, there are some playful things you can do with a foreskin if your partner is willing.

DID YOU KNOW?

Worldwide, about a quarter of all males are circumcised. Circumcision is an ancient practice that is religiously prescribed for Muslims and Jews. Now it is also practiced as a religious and nonreligious tradition in many countries.

Gentle Tugging

Gently pull the foreskin above the head of the penis with one hand, then place the thumb and forefinger of your other hand on opposite sides of the corona (See Appendix A - Anatomy for location details). Let go of the foreskin with one hand as you move your thumb and forefinger in quick up and down motions over the head, or try rotating and twisting your fingers at the same time. Alternatively, pull the foreskin above the head of the penis with one hand and then wrap your other hand (all five fingers) around the base of the penis while you move it in circular or up and down motions.

The Turkey Baster

Take a turkey baster or ear syringe and fill it with warm water. Gently pull the foreskin over the head of the penis and lightly pinch it over the tip of the baster. Fill the foreskin with the warm water then release the bulb of the baster in order to suck the water back up. Do this once—or quickly over and over again—for a pulsating sensation almost like a warm vibration.

DID YOU KNOW?

Some groups—such as The Canadian Foreskin Awareness Project—are on a crusade to stop circumcision and have made it their life goal to educate the public on its adverse effects. This feisty pro-foreskin advocacy group promotes foreskin education, appreciation and stimulation. In some countries however circumcision is still deemed important to curtail the spread of disease. In the western world, proper cleaning/grooming practices have helped minimize transmission therefore making circumcision for these purposes unnecessary.

Shower Head

Gently pull the foreskin over the head of the penis and open it up slightly, almost like forming a small basket or bucket. Using a retractable shower head, angle it so the water squirts directly into the penis (being mindful of the water pressure and temperature). While you shower your partner's penis with wonderful water sensations, you may want to spend some time upping the visuals—by lathering yourself with bubble bath—or take your partner's clean testes in your mouth while kneeling in the shower.

Remember to always treat the foreskin with care. Pulling on the foreskin too aggressively, or in haste before your partner has become fully aroused can cause ripping or tearing.

10

Who Said You Shouldn't Play With Your Food?!

The possibilities are endless when it comes to adding edible and tasty add-ons to your oral fixation, however be mindful of too much contact with anything too extreme—too hot, too cold, too spicy, etc.—as the penis is a very sensitive organ. That said, everything in moderation opens the floodgates for fun. Unlike females, most males do not have the same risk factors for yeast infections, so sugary treats are more than ok. Just be careful that nothing gets left behind under the foreskin - if your partner is uncircumcised—and wipe them down or wash them off thoroughly before intercourse, particularly if you are female bodied.

Common fun foods include honey, jam, whipped cream, melted/liquid chocolate, and ice cream. Or if you are the adventurous type, the Smell and Taste Research Foundation in Chicago found that various smells can increase penile blood flow, such as: pumpkin pie, licorice, donuts, lavender, oriental spice, and cola (See Chapter 5 for tips on *Setting the Stage*). A cleverly hung donut can therefore serve a dual purpose, adding a bit of sweetness for you and little something to get your partner's blood flowing as they watch you get your fill.

For a more visual experience you can slowly and sensually lick a Popsicle and then use your cold tongue, or the Popsicle itself, to tease and trace their penis. Your partner will probably never look at the summer treat the same way again. You could also try placing a small marshmallow in each side of your cheek while your partner penetrates your mouth. This should allow a smooth, tight, and sticky sensation.

The tried and true breath mint or cough drop, stealthily placed in your mouth just prior to providing oral sex, can add sensations ranging from tingly and terrific to numbing and painful (depending on brand and exposure amount. Always check with your partner first). You can also try placing a dab of toothpaste in your mouth before inserting the penis for a quick freshness and tingle on both ends.The ideas for penis-to-food combos are endless, as it's pretty safe to say that if you can eat it, you can bring it to the party. Play around with a variety of types and brands, as finding the perfect product that you both enjoy— with no burning, itching, or stinging sensations—is half the battle and half the fun. And don't forget, eating anything that you enjoy (whether it's at the dinner table or in the bedroom) can be made into something that's sensual, sexy, and fun. The possibilities are limited only by your imagination and preferences.

THE GRAPEFRUIT – THE BREAKFAST OF CHAMPIONS

Preparing the grapefruit

Make sure the fruit is at room temperature or slightly warmer. To warm it slightly, simply put the fruit in warm water for a few minutes (do not microwave or boil it). Then roll the fruit back and forth for 10-20 seconds on a hard desk or counter; this rolling technique juices the grapefruit up just slightly. Next, find the two navels located on either side of the fruit. Place the grapefruit on a plate and cut off both ends—where the navels are located—so that the fruit would sit level on a table without rolling around. Then cut out a hole in the grapefruit that is roughly the size of your partner's penis (don't make it too big and don't make it too tight). Make sure the hole goes straight through the fruit so you can see through the grapefruit from one side to the other.

DID YOU KNOW?

A grapefruit is also a fat burner so you are actually losing weight while giving oral sex.

Game time

Once your partner is erect and raring to go then place the grapefruit over the penis. Hold the fruit in one hand and go up and down the shaft with it. However don't stop using your mouth, as you can focus the fruit on the base and use your suction and tongue techniques on the tip or head of the penis at the same time. Mix it up by twisting the fruit from side to side and squeezing it slightly in conjunction with the up and down motions of your mouth. If a grapefruit is too large, you can also use a navel orange.

DID YOU KNOW?

There is a published semen cookbook called Natural Harvest —A collection of Semen Based Recipes (cookingwithcum.com). The author proclaims: "Semen is not only nutritious, but it also has a wonderful texture and amazing cooking properties. Like fine wine and cheeses, the taste of semen is complex and dynamic. Semen is an exciting ingredient that can give every dish you make an interesting twist. If you are a passionate cook and are not afraid to experiment with new ingredients—you will love this cook book!" The Gourmand World Cookbook Award nominated book does deliver a plethora of recipes and tips for cooking with semen. However the question isn't so much why someone would want to cook with semen, but rather how consistent is it as an ingredient? Some semen is quite acidic while other semen is rather sweet; sweet is, of course, a relative term. So can you really trust the ingredient to taste as the chef intended it to? Or will each of these recipes be dependent on the donors' lifestyle?

PART TWO:
BEYOND THE BLOW JOB

11

Nonsense and Other Tall Tales

It's not a good blow job if you can't deep throat – Bullshit

The most sensitive part of the penis is the head and surrounding area (such as the frenulum), the least sensitive for most males, is the base of the penis. Therefore if you can't get your gums over the entire penis, don't stress. Many people don't find the deep throat to be their orgasm trigger anyways.

If a male doesn't get hard right away they are not enjoying themselves – Bullshit

Some people take awhile to get hard—especially as they age—but that doesn't mean that every lick, kiss, and touch from you doesn't feel amazing, and that they are not completely and utterly turned on by you. Many individuals love watching a penis get hard in front of them, feeling it grow inside their mouth over time. Others prefer their partners to be hard before they venture down below. Either way, try not to doubt your attractiveness and/or abilities if your partner isn't fully erect in minutes.

It's not great head if you don't swallow – Bullshit

Some people do prefer to finish where they've started, in your warm enticing mouth. It's an easy clean up (just a swallow away from tidy) and there are often no breaks between what was leading them up to an orgasm and the actually finale. However some people prefer their partners don't swallow so they can see their ejaculate.

If your partner doesn't ejaculate then they didn't have an orgasm – Bullshit

Yes, in most cases an orgasm does go hand-in-hand with an ejaculation, however these two functions do not have to be combined. Some people can control the release of their ejaculate until they see fit, which may be after two or more orgasms. A combination of strong PC muscles (which can be strengthened through Kegel exercises) and many hours of practise to learn when to contract these muscles, is key. If squeezed at the right moment during arousal, an orgasm can occur without the release of ejaculate.

There is also a condition called Retrograde Ejaculation. This condition results in an orgasm without semen release outside the body. Instead of ejaculate being released through the urethral, it is released into the bladder.

It's all about the money shot – Bullshit

Not ejaculating does not mean that someone is an inferior lover. It is important to not equate success with ejaculation, as it should be more about the process than the final result. They call it forePLAY for a reason, therefore taking the goals out of your intimacy interactions is the first step towards pleasure filled enjoyment. This is especially important as your partner gets older and may not be able to ejaculate as easily. By not focusing solely on "the money shot" as a measure of success, one can reduce the amount of pressure an individual may feel to reach climax, as this can cause a lot of anxiety and disappointment surrounding sex and ones self image, on both sides.

Sperm is good for your skin therefore you should get a "facial" to conclude each blow job – Bullshit

Sperm facials: Professionals use a synthesized version of spermine to soothe and moisturize the face, treat sun damage and diminish wrinkles. Spermine, not to be confused with semen, is a robust antioxidant, and while present in seminal fluid in small quantities, it's also found in human skin cells. Therefore, you are better off using a traditional moisturizer instead of counting on the small quantities of spermine present in semen to give you a youthful glow.

If your partner is not hard, they can't ejaculate – Bullshit

Male-bodied individuals can and do ejaculate while flaccid. In fact many males experience this regardless of their age or sexual health.

DID YOU KNOW?

Mating pairs of Sepia officinalis (most commonly known as Cuttle-fish) align their bodies head to head while mating so the male can transfer a sealed package of sperm into a pouch just beneath the female's mouth. The female then scurries off to a quiet place where she draws eggs from her cavity and then passes them over the sperm, thereby fertilising them. In the event of there being multiple sperm deposits, it is the one at the back of the queue, i.e. the last to deposit near this mouth cavity, who takes the title of proud poppa.

12

Common Concerns and FAQ's

I really don't want to perform oral sex on my partner. Is there something wrong with me?

First off: It's only a problem if you feel it's a problem. If it truly doesn't bother you or your partner that oral sex is not a part of your relationship, congratulations—you are fine!

Secondly, if you currently don't want to engage in oral sex, but would like this to change, let's take a step back from the actual act and look at the relationship as a whole: How is your communication? Are you feeling heard and respected? Are you feeling hurt and angry? Are you feeling shamed or pressured? Is there something happening within the relationship that doesn't fit with your morals or values? Are you feeling suspicious that there are secrets or lies between you and your partner? How is your partner's hygiene? Is there a smell or situation that is unappealing to you? There are many factors that could be contributing to you not wanting to engage in oral sex and again, they are very common. Effective, respectful communication can usually address these concerns and clear the way to eliminating these barriers.

Now if you have gone through the relationship piece by piece and you truly can't find any reason blocking you from participating and you still want to try oral sex, you may look into speaking with a professional to help you uncover what is blocking you from moving forward. Common emotional and subconscious reasons could include: beliefs that it is bad or wrong, a worry around STIs/STDs, past trauma or abuse, among many others.

Moral of the story, you are fine just the way you are; however, if you would like to change, there are resources available to help you do so.

I'm afraid I'm going to hurt my partner's penis. How will I know how much pressure is enough or too much?

Short answer—ask your partner. Just like people, no two penises are the same; some can handle a lot of pressure, some need a delicate touch. If you are unsure about the kind of grip, pressure, or pleasure points that your partner likes, ask them to take you for a hand ride.

What is a hand ride you say? We would be more than happy to tell you...

Place your hand on your partner's penis, and then they place their hand over yours and guide you with the exact placement, pressure, and pace that fans their fire. Alternatively, you can place your hand over your partner's as they guide you to their own personal bliss. This can be a handy exercise for the entire body to get a sense of one's personal hot spots and will no doubt be educational and bonding for you both.

My partner's penis points straight down when it is erect, is that normal?

Although many people assume a penis should align horizontally with the floor when standing erect, many penises point north, south, east or west—this is perfectly normal.

What's really in ejaculate?

Many people believe that their semen is a tasty non-dairy treat that is meant to be savoured and enjoyed. And according to most mainstream pornography, every partner not only agrees, but they fall to their knees in avid anticipation for this tasty treat. Fact or fiction? You be the judge.

Ejaculate may not be as tasty as porn leads us to believe, but it may contain a few ingredients that aren't half bad. Semen, or seminal fluid, is a thick, off-white liquid ejaculated from the urethra which can coincide with sexual climax. Sperm only account for approximately 1% of the total volume of the semen, with a single ejaculation usually ranging between 2-5 millilitres (1 tsp), and containing between 100-700 million sperm.

Side note: According to research, the average sperm counts in several Western countries dropped by nearly one-half between 1940-1990. A drop in ejaculate volume was also detected. Environmental toxins have been suspected to have contributed to this wide spreading effect on sperm in the US, Canada, and other countries over the last several decades.

So, if sperm only account for 1% of the semen, where does the other 99% of the seminal fluid come from? As mentioned earlier, a large portion comes from the seminal vesicles and the prostate gland, and less than 1% comes from the testes. And within this mixture, there is a large degree of fructose (sugar), calcium binders (citric acid), enzymes, vitamins and antioxidants. We'd list all the ingredients in semen however it has more than 300 constituents (including proteins, fats, immature sperm cells, dead parts of sperm, and occasionally blood cells).

Why does semen sometimes leave a yellowish stain on towels/cloths?

Semen contains protein (mostly albumin) which is the same kind of protein that is in egg whites. As protein dries it changes colour. Males with a lower volume ejaculate containing many white blood cells may leave a more yellowish semen stain on garments as the protein dries.

Why does it hurt so bad when I get semen in my eye?

Testicle fluid and sperm are odourless, however the seminal vesicles and the prostate add an odour to semen that many would characterize as a cleaning product smell. This sometimes intense aroma is from spermine (which is made by the prostate). Spermine is a member of the chemical family known as polyamines, which can have a corrosive effect. Now the concentration of spermine in ejaculate isn't nearly as high as its pure chemical form, however it's no wonder that a little slash to the eye can cause a burning sensation. If an accident does happen however, rinsing your eye with water should do the trick.

DID YOU KNOW?

The testicles are not completely symmetrical. One testicle (most often the left) hangs lower, and one (usually the right), is slightly larger.

The skin on the shaft of my partner's penis is a lot darker than the skin around the rest of their body, is that normal?

The skin tone on your partner might be quite different than the skin tone on their penis, and that's perfectly normal. The skin covering your partner's penis may be darker or lighter than the rest of their body; similarly, they may have freckles, spots, or blotches that appear only on their shaft or scrotum.

DID YOU KNOW?

If you are holding back from letting your partner ejaculate in your mouth because you can't stand the taste, there is a product called Masque™ Sexual Flavors, an orally dissolube flavoured strip that sits on your tongue and is meant to mask the taste of semen. The 3 Strip Wallet Pack is available in four different flavours: mango, strawberry, watermelon, and chocolate. The company claims that the taste-masking ingredients remain active for up to fifteen minutes and finish with a cool, minty note. Each gel strip is packaged individually with a foil wrap, ensuring freshness for the length of shelf life.

Is semen an antidepressant?

Researchers have found that women who had partners that did not use condoms scored lower on tests for depression than women who had partners that did use condoms; and women who had partners that were using condoms, showed similar amounts of depression to women who weren't having intercourse at all. Research also showed that women who had most recently received a semen deposit had the lowest levels of depression among all subjects who were tested. Studies such as these have lead researchers to believe that the hormones in semen are actually absorbed into a female's body through their vagina, and that these hormones do have an anti-depressive or mood-elevating effect.

It should be noted that the authors of these studies looked for other factors that could explain the differences in depression level between women (such as length of relationship, birth-control pills, high-risk sexual behaviour vs. low-risk sexual behaviours, etc.) however, none of these could explain the differences in the female's mood. Now although these findings are preliminary, they do suggest a relationship between vaginal semen intake and depression. Perhaps semen has more positive benefits than once thought.

There is no research—that we have found—linking swallowing semen and antidepressant effects on men or women.

Is it possible to be allergic to semen?

Yes. Semen allergies are caused by an allergic reaction to a particular protein in semen. Symptoms include a burning and itching feeling that often occurs wherever the semen comes into contact with the body, such as the mouth, stomach, anus, and vagina. To determine if you are experiencing a semen allergy try using condoms for a few weeks (you may want to use polyurethane condoms as you could also be experiencing a reaction to latex). If the symptoms appear only after non-condom usage then it's time to make an appointment with your doctor. If you are having an allergic reaction to semen there is a desensitizing treatment that is safe and effective; switching mates however, is not going to help. If you suddenly become allergic to one partner's ejaculate, you will generally be allergic to all ejaculate.

What is smegma?

Smegma is produced, and collected under, the foreskin in males and around the clitoris and in the folds of the labia in females. It is said that smegma helps keep the glands moist (for facilitating intercourse), however most males and females prefer its absence to its presence. An odour can accompany noticeable smegma, which is whitish in colour, however the substance — caused by the shedding of skin cells—is relatively harmless (unless it's allowed to build up). When good (and recent) hygiene is being practiced, smegma is not a common sight.

What if my partner doesn't cum at all, is that normal?

This can either be looked at as a blessing, or a curse. Some individuals simply do not ejaculate from oral sex. This doesn't have to be a reflection on a partner's sexual skills or techniques. In order to have future fellatio go smoothly, speak to your partner about an appropriate length of time for performing a blow job. Constant reassurance about the giver's abilities, as well as good vocalization on the pleasure being obtained during, can be beneficial.

DID YOU KNOW?

Research shows that individuals prefer equality when comparing themselves to their partners, but prefer superiority when comparing themselves to other couples. So at the end of the day, many people claim they are happiest when they feel their relationship is seen as better than people in comparable relationships

Can the penis actually be broken or sprained?

Although a "pop" or cracking sound has been reported when a male's erection was suddenly bent in a way that nature didn't intend, no bone is actually present in the human penis, therefore nothing could be broken in the literal sense of the word. That being said, if a penis is subjected to this kind of unfortunate and painful bending, the owner of said penis should get to a hospital right away. A popping sound could be an indication that a ligament in the penis has snapped; this could cause internal bleeding, which can result in permanent damage to the penis. Waiting more than a few hours to seek help is unwise.

A penis can also develop Peyronie's disease if it is continuously bent or tweaked. This disease—believed to be caused by patches of calcium collecting on these twisted and pinched penile areas—causes bent and sometimes painful erections. Peyronie's is also not easy to treat and can cause long-term disfigurement.

It is important to note that any penial pain that lasts more than 10-15 minutes needs to be addressed immediately by a medical professional. Don't wait simply because you may be embarrassed to seek help, as long-term disfigurement and erectile pain is a far worse position to be in.

DID YOU KNOW?

In cats, dogs, and many other mammals, males have a penis-stiffening bone called the 'os pubis.' In the walrus this bony support is nearly as long as a man's arm. This brings a whole new meaning to the term boner.

13

Research

Some of the most frequently asked questions we hear as sex therapists are: What's normal? What are other people doing? Am I doing this enough? Am I doing this too much? Am I the only person who's into that? Among many others...

So why is everyone asking the same types of questions, especially when it comes to sex? The reason is a little something called the Social Comparison Theory that was developed by social psychologist Leon Festinger in 1954. The theory states that if there is no objective standard that can be used as a benchmark, we compare ourselves to others to decide if we are ok with where we stand. So for example, if someone gets an A on a test, they know they did well even if they were the only person who took the exam, but if someone is turned on sexually by something, because it is a personal experience that can't actually be measured, we often look to other people's experiences of arousal and rank our experiences against theirs to decide if we're "normal."

We're more likely to use social comparison when we are stressed, don't know what to expect, or are feeling vulnerable. And what is more vulnerable that being naked and intimate with another person? Nowhere to hide there! And we don't compare ourselves against just anybody. We often like to compare ourselves to people we consider "just like us" instead of those who we think are different. And why do we do that? Because we want to compare apples to apples instead of apples to oranges.

So how do these comparisons impact us? If we feel that we are doing "worse" than others we are likely unhappy, and if we feel we are doing "better" we are likely pretty satisfied. We tend to view the world like this when we are uncertain of our own self-worth in a situation, or don't have really clear internal standards. Sex is so subjective it can be difficult to feel confident, so we look to what others are doing to reassure ourselves. However, research has found that people who frequently focus on these comparisons to others versus looking inside themselves to determine satisfaction tend to be generally less happy overall. So the old saying actually is true; happiness really does start from within (but apparently we still secretly like to be better than our friends).

This idea of social comparison in sexual relationships inspired one of us to do some research and explore the impact that sexual frequency had on relationship satisfaction and sexual satisfaction.

Over 200 participants filled out an anonymous online survey, filling out scales measuring current sexual satisfaction and relationship satisfaction and noting the variety and frequency of sexual acts. Participants were then asked how often they would have sex/oral sex, how often they wanted sex/oral sex, how often they thought they should be having it, and how often they thought other people were having it.

The biggest predictor of satisfaction was not what participants were actually doing, but what they were doing in comparison to what they thought other people were doing. For example, if people were participating in oral sex once per week but thought other people were doing it four times per week, they tended to have lower relationship and sexual satisfaction and vice versa. It brings whole new meaning to the phrase "keeping up with the Joneses." Having more frequent sexual activity than the people they compared themselves to was even more predictive of sexual satisfaction than if what they were doing lined up with what they desired or felt they should be doing sexually.

So what does this research mean for you? Chances are your sexual satisfaction is linked to how you feel you compare to your friends or others around you (and definitely Hollywood). However it is likely they are exaggerating how great their sex lives are.

Check in with yourself. Who are you comparing yourself to and is that realistic? Are you taking your own wants and needs into the equation? Is that comparison helping or hurting you?

Your sex life is yours to create and explore. It is personal, and tailor-made for you, by you. Comparing your sex life to someone else's is often a misinformed and a surefire way to feel bad about your own sex life. If you and your partner are happy—you're fine. Go forth and be awesome; quit worrying about what everyone else says they are doing.

DID YOU KNOW?

When two flatworms of one oceanic species meet, a sex fight generally follows. All flatworms are hermaphrodites (they have both male and female sex organs), so each has a penis and uses the device like a hypodermic needle—trying to pierce the other with it. As one lunges the other dodges and strikes back. Imagine penis fencing! This fight can last an hour before one flatworm makes a hit, injecting sperm into the other, anywhere along the body. The winner then swims off in triumph.

14

Sometimes It's Not All Fun And Games

Some of you picked up this book to fuel your curiosity and add to your ever-expanding repertoire between the sheets. For others, the idea of sticking a penis in your mouth is enough to induce a panic attack. If you find your experience of oral sex closer to the latter, here are some suggestions that may help you understand your fears and decide a course of action that fits for you.

A PICTURE IS WORTH A THOUSAND WORDS

In some cases there may be anxiety around what you are going to find below the belt, and this can show up for a variety of reasons. The first of which being: not having a penis or never taking anyone else's for a test drive. In other words, a lack of personal experience. If your goal is to get comfortable with giving blow jobs, you are going to have to get really comfortable with penises. So your first assignment is...drumroll please...find some penis pictures and check them out.

DID YOU KNOW?

A draft from the California Division of Occupational Safety and Health (OSHA) is putting forward bill AB640, which is a 21-page draft that would require actors to wear safety goggles (and condoms) on porn shoots by law. The OSHA claims goggles will avoid semen from entering the eyes, a body part susceptible to diseases such as HIV and Chlamydia (November 2013).

Now be warned, if you go to Google and just type in 'penis', you are going to see things you can never un-see (often in the "should I see a doctor about this?" category). Again you have been warned. Ideally find a reputable source that shows you a variety of pictures—circumcised or non-circumcised, hard or flaccid. This way you can get up-close and personal without being up-close and personal to see what "generally" you're working with. Remember, no two penises are alike but at least you will have a basic idea.

ARE YOUR FEARS GETTING IN THE WAY

Next, write out any fears and anxieties you may have about blow jobs. When you know what you're worried about then you can work towards overcoming those fears.

Some common ones are:

- I think it will smell or semen will taste bad.
- I'm afraid I will choke.
- I'm afraid I might throw up.
- I'm afraid I'll get lockjaw.
- I'm afraid my partner will grab the back of my head.
- I'm afraid its wrong.
- I'm afraid I'll be judged.

Once you've identified your roadblocks, depending on what they are, you may want to try one of the following exercises:

BOUNDARIES

If your fears are based around logistical concerns such as being grabbed or choking, this is a great time to start using your words and create some boundaries that work for you. Remember, you get to decide what you do with your body and with your partner. You decide what you're comfortable with, but it is also your responsibility to let your partner know what you are and aren't okay with. If you aren't okay with them touching your head, let them know that is a no-go zone. If you're not on board with swallowing semen, let your partner know they need to give you lots of notice before they are about to ejaculate so you can pull away and use your hand, or so they can finish themselves off. It's always a negotiation.

If taste is a concern, you can ask that you both take a shower first, or use a flavoured lube. Check in with your partner and talk about what you are both comfortable with.

BABY STEPS

If you are worried about gagging or lockjaw, or are apprehensive in general, start with baby steps. Don't think that you are going to just go from nothing to deep-throating (remember: not everybody does that). Start small. Maybe just spend some time kissing your partner's penis, then licking it. See how that feels. You may then decide to place just the tip of their penis in your mouth. Again, it's whatever you are comfortable with. You decide how far you want to go.

VALUES CLASH

If you find that the reason you are uncomfortable with blow jobs is because it's in conflict with a value system—yours, your family's, your religion's, or your culture's—we recommend speaking to a professional who can help you make peace with your choices and support you in deciding what fits for you.

HOW TO TALK TO YOUR PARTNER ABOUT ORAL SEX

Remember, it starts with you.

You need to get clear on what you are or are not comfortable with. What are you interested in? What turns you on? What is too much for you? Where are the boundaries of what you are comfortable with?

Once you know where you stand, you can then look at communicating this to your partner(s).

Use "I" Language

Speak about your own feelings, needs, and experiences from your own perspective without blaming.

Use clear language

Be specific about what you need or prefer. Focus on your feelings, wants, and desires, as opposed to what the other person is or isn't doing.

Try something like:

"I feel really turned on when we shower together. I would love it if we had more showers together because it really gets me in the mood."

Try the sandwich technique

If there is a difficult conversation you need to address, try the sandwich technique—something positive, something difficult, something positive.

For example: [positive] I get turned on when you walk around without a shirt on and make the effort to set the mood before oral sex. However, [negative] sometimes when you grab the back of my head, and push my face towards your penis, it makes me feel uncomfortable and a bit disrespected. [positive] I feel that if you tapped my shoulders instead of grabbing my head, I would get the idea of what you wanted and would be more excited about going down on you. I do love watching you climax while I'm on my knees though, and I think this would help me feel more comfortable and more turned on.

IS YOUR RELATIONSHIP THE PROBLEM?

One thing that you should consider if you find yourself apprehensive or unsure about oral sex is this - is your anxiety trying to tell you something about your relationship? Sometimes our bodies can raise the alarm when there is something not right between us and our partners that needs to be addressed. Ask yourself: do you feel comfortable discussing concerns with your partner? Do you feel like your needs and boundaries are being respected? Do you feel like you can trust your partner? Do you feel like you are being pressured to do something you are not comfortable with? True sexual intimacy involves being vulnerable, and that can only be achieved if you feel safe with your partner. If you're not feeling safe, there may be other issues that need to be addressed before you can work on the sexual side of your relationship.

ARE YOUR BELIEFS HOLDING YOU BACK?

Sometimes we can have beliefs about sex and sexuality that can get in the way of us fully expressing our sexual selves. The problem is we often don't know what beliefs we hold until we stop and take the time to explore. The following exercise and questions are designed to help you gain a greater understanding of yourself and your beliefs around sex and sexuality.

Sexual Timeline

Get a large piece of paper and place it lengthwise in front of you. Draw a line across the middle of the paper and at one end label it birth or 0 and at the other end label it present or your current age. Then place a small line or dot on the line for each year of your life. Depending on your current age you may need to use more than one piece of paper.

Under the line, write out any significant life events or stressors as they correspond to the various years/ages on your timeline. These can be things like moving, switching schools, graduating, getting married, getting new jobs, any illnesses or injuries, etc. Over the line, start writing out any significant events regarding your sexuality or other events that would have impacted your sexuality. For example: when you first heard about sex, first kiss, first sexual touch, first intercourse, any relationships, negative sexual interactions, positive sexual revelations, and if female – first period and/or pregnancies, births, or abortions..

For some people, doing this exercise can bring up uncomfortable memories and emotions. Alternatively, for some it can be very liberating and empowering. If disturbing feelings arise for you, we recommend that you seek out support from a professional or someone you trust.

Once you have completed the timeline take a step back: What do you notice? Are there any patterns or themes that you can see? Any direct correlations or connections between events? Did anything surprise you? Does anything feel clearer to you?

Questions to Ponder

- How did you first learn about sex and in particular, oral sex?
- Was it accurate information?
- As you grew up, was intercourse and oral sex embraced as healthy and normal, dirty and shameful, or something in between?
- Were you ever forced or coerced to perform sexual acts that you didn't want to?

- What were your family beliefs around sex?
  - What were you told about sex and oral sex?
  - Under what circumstances was it OK?
  - Under what circumstances was it not OK?
  - Was there open conversation or was it something left unsaid?

There can be many reasons that oral sex can be an uncomfortable topic or act to approach—some logistical, some rooted deeply in your subconscious. We want to stress that what you do or do not do with your partner/s is a personal choice and you have the right to decide what fits for you. If you find yourself struggling, we recommend that you seek out a certified professional in your area to guide and support you.

DID YOU KNOW?

Ejaculate can sometimes smell of household cleaning products (such as Clorox). The fluid produced by the testes and the semen itself however, are in fact odourless. The smell comes from the portion of ejaculate produced by the seminal vesicles and the prostate gland.

15

Giving – Receiving – Allowing – Taking

There are different kinds of sexual energy and each contains value and benefits for both partners. It can be interesting to explore which aspects of these energies feel more comfortable for you, for your partner, and if there is a pattern that you find yourself in. You may also want to try to develop areas you are less skilled in so that you can become a more well-rounded sexual being, giving you more options for pleasurable sexual expression.

Other Focused	Self Focused
Giving	Receiving
Allowing	Taking

GIVING

Giving energy is a selfless energy where the focus is on your partner. It is giving of pleasure, giving of self, and other-focused. Performing oral sex can be a very giving act as the personal pleasure is coming more from the pleasure you are giving to your partner, instead of actual personal physical arousal. (Performing oral sex can be in the taking category if you enjoy doing it.)

Giving can be expressed in asking the question: How would you like to be touched (for your pleasure)?

ALLOWING

Allowing energy is also an other-focused energy. Although you are the recipient, you are allowing your partner to give to you. For example: after a fight, some people enjoy giving their partner sexual pleasure or receiving sexual closeness as a way to help deal with the anxiety of the conflict. Allowing your partner to be sexually close to you (as long as you feel comfortable with it) can be a very healing experience, even if the focus is not on pleasure.

Allowing can be expressed in asking the question: How would you like to touch me (for your pleasure)?

RECEIVING

Receiving energy is a self-focused energy where you are focused on the pleasure you are receiving from a sexual act instead of focusing on reciprocating.

Receiving can be expressed in answering the question: How would I like to be touched (for my pleasure)?

TAKING

Taking energy is one in which you are the dominant—using your partner for your own pleasure. It can be a very raw and intense energy and depending on your partner, quite pleasurable for them as well.

Taking can be expressed in answering the question: How would you like to touch me (for my pleasure)?

The reality is that there is pleasure in all of the quadrants and gifts in all of them:

Giving - generosity, being of service to another

Receiving - gratitude, expressing what you want

Taking - responsibility, not taking more than is offered, being shamelessly selfish

Allowing - surrender, letting go of having to be in control

Of course for all of this to work it has to happen with consent no matter what quadrant you're in.

GIVING-RECEIVING-ALLOWING-TAKING was adapted from the Wheel of Consent by Dr. Betty Martin www.bettymartin.org.

THE HAPPY ENDING

There is no way that we could even begin to contain the range of what is possible in one book. So please do not take this book as the gospel on oral sex, instead see it as a place to start.

We hope this book got the juices flowing both literally and figuratively, and you continue on this journey of discovery.

Appendix A - Anatomy

Knowing Your Instrument

There is a What?! Where?!

We are aware that there are always a few people that will scoff at the need for this section, assured that there isn't much to the penis and testes. However, what these folks may not know is that there are many important parts to this organ that lie beneath the surface; parts that some find hard to pronounce, and others that you may not even know existed. So sit down, relax and get ready for this quick rundown of what you're dealing with.

THE FACTS

The mean (or average) penile length for a non-erect penis is approximately 9.3 +/- 1.3 cm (around 3.5 inches) and the mean penile circumference for a non-erect penis is approximately 9.31 cm (around 3.6 inches). The mean length of an erect penis is approximately 13.7 +/- 1.6 cm (around 5.5 inches) and the mean penile circumference of an erect penis is approximately 11.66 cm (around 4.6 inches). There also seems to be a weak, but positive, correlation found between penile length and a male's height, weight, and body mass index. What that means is that if you run into a giant, chances are he will be equipped with a larger than average tool; however, just because an individual is large or small doesn't necessarily mean their penis will follow suit.

The figures on what is considered to be a "normal" penis size can be misleading and disheartening for many, as feeling inadequate can have devastating psychological effects. Some turn away from the possibility of intimacy due to embarrassment, while others turn to augmentation surgery or liposuction. Some male-bodied individuals feel as though their flaccid penis retracts inside their bodies, decreasing the overall length of the penis. However this can be a consequence of obesity, as the prepubic fat pad may become so thick and large that the flaccid penis is barely long enough to protrude through it. Weight loss may alleviate this problem. The surgical means of penis lengthening often includes the cutting of the suspensory ligament (followed by many weeks of traction—hanging weights from the penis). Other men try and increase their girth through fat injections, or by transplanting slabs of fatty tissue from the buttocks to the penis. The flip side of these expensive surgeries is that the men who request them typically have average-sized penises and are usually dissatisfied with the outcome. To top it off, they do not report experiencing an improvement in their sex lives afterwards.

So what does all this penile augmentation talk have to do with you? It highlights an important and highly sensitive topic. Just because your partner may fall above or below the average statistic, it doesn't mean that they are any better or worse a lover, or that their penis can't provide more than enough pleasure for every orifice of your body. In fact, a smaller than average penis will work to your benefit for both oral and anal sex, and depending on the curvature of your partner's penis, a smaller curved package may be better for hitting that elusive G-Spot in females.

But we digress.

Let's get back to the nitty-gritty of this chapter: The anatomy of the penis. When looking at the male external genitals in their natural form, a.k.a. uncircumcised or intact, you will see two distinct portions: the penis (shaft) and the scrotum (balls). Now to avoid becoming too technical, let us give you the quick version of what's inside these organs.

DID YOU KNOW?

Delusions of penile retraction have swept across some Asian countries from time to time. This condition is known as Koro. Those inflicted often attach clamps, strings and other devices to their penis in order to prevent its complete disappearance, which they are convinced will be followed by their own death.

THE PENIS: SHAFT

On the outside of the shaft you will find the head (or glans), the corona, the frenulum, the urethral orifice, and the foreskin. On the inside of the shaft you will find the corpora cavernosa, corpora spongiosum, and the urethra.

HEAD OR GLANS

The glans is the bulbous section near the tip of the penis and can be highly sensitive, particularly in uncircumcised men and is usually covered by the prepuce unless the penis is erect or the male is circumcised.

DID YOU KNOW?

The Kama Sutra gives a detailed account on how to enlarge one's penis. It is to be accomplished by repeated application of the bristles of certain tree living insects, followed by rubbing the penis with oil for 10 nights and sleeping with the penis hanging down through a hole in the bed. If this "lengthening" procedure does not provide their partner with pleasure and satisfaction, the Kama Sutra advises that the male use apadravyas (which are metal or ivory sleeves studded with "pleasure bumps" on the outside). These fit over the penis in a modular fashion, increasing both its girth and length as much as the male, or their partner, desires. If there is an extreme case of minute penis size, the book recommends that the male forget about the penis altogether and simply tie the tubular stalk of a bottle gourd around his waist with a string. This will create a version of what has come to be known as a strap-on dildo.

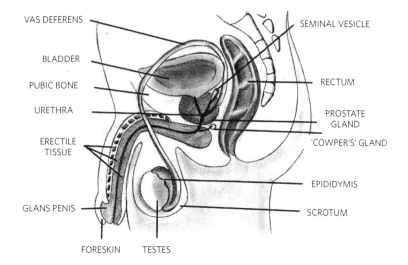

VAS DEFERENS

SEMINAL VESICLE

BLADDER

PUBIC BONE

RECTUM

URETHRA

PROSTATE
GLAND

ERECTILE
TISSUE

'COWPER'S' GLAND

EPIDIDYMIS

GLANS PENIS

SCROTUM

FORESKIN   TESTES

CORONA

Connects the glans to the shaft of the penis. Corona, meaning the 'crown,' is a ridge of flesh where the head of the penis and the shaft join.

FRENULUM

Located on the underside of the penis where the corona makes a V shape. It can often be seen by locating the thin strip of flesh on the underside of the penis that connects the shaft to the head. Although stimulation anywhere on the penis can be sexually arousing, the corona and the frenulum are usually the most erotically sensitive regions. (See the Tips and Techniques section under "Focusing on the Frenulum" for a diagram of this area)

URETHRAL ORIFICE (OR URETHRAL MEATUS)

The opening most commonly found (although not always) at the center of the tip of the penis to allow the passage of both urine and semen.

PREPUCE / FORESKIN

In uncircumcised males you will see a loose, tubular fold of skin referred to as the prepuce, or more commonly, the foreskin, which can partially or fully cover the glans while the penis is flaccid. The foreskin is very rich in nerve endings. Circumcision is the name of the procedure that surgically removes the foreskin.

CORPORA CAVERNOSA AND CORPORA SPONGIOSUM

The shaft of the penis contains three erectile structures: two corpora cavernosa and a thinner corpus spongiosum. The corpora cavernosa accounts for the bulk of the penis's erectile capacity. Both of these structures extend backward into the body, forming the root of the penis.

URETHRA

Discharges urine from the bladder and semen from the reproductive glands.

THE SCROTUM/SCROTAL SAC: BALLS

The scrotum is a sac that hangs behind and below the penis and contains the testes (testicles). The scrotum's primary function is to maintain the testes at an optimal temperature. The production of sperm, for example, requires a range of 4-7°C below core body temperature. This is why the testicles are on the outside of the body and why you will sometimes notice the scrotum tighten (to heat up) and loosen (to cool down) as the body regulates the testicles' temperature.

On the outside of the scrotum you will find a light covering of hair and numerous sweat glands that help to regulate the temperature of the testicles. Simplistically speaking, on the inside of the scrotum you will find the testes, the epididymis and the vas deferens.

DID YOU KNOW?

A condition known as hypospadias is the product of the urethral folds failing to fully enclose the urethra. This results in the urethra opening at different areas of the penis: such as on the shaft of the penis, at the base of the penis, on the front of the scrotum, or even on the perineum behind the testicles. It is estimated that hypospadias (severe enough to require surgical repair) occurs in as many as 1 in 350 boys; however, far greater numbers present with milder forms.

TESTES

The testes (weighing approximately 10-15 grams) have two distinct functions: they produce sperm and secrete sex hormones.

EPIDIDYMIS

This structure takes the form of the letter C and is attached to the back surface of the testes. Sperm spend about a week traversing through this, during which time they become far more concentrated and functionally mature, which gives them the capacity for forward swimming motions. This structure is where the sperm pass through after leaving the testes.

VAS DEFERENS

Conveys mature sperm away from the epididymis and contains arteries, veins, and nerves that supply each testicle.

PROSTATE GLAND

A single chestnut-sized gland located immediately below the bladder. The secretion of the prostate is a cloudy alkaline fluid. This gland produces approximately 30% of the total volume of ejaculate.

SEMINAL VESICLES

These glands produce approximately 70% of the total volume of ejaculate, however their name is misleading as they are not storage areas for the semen. As with the prostate, the fluid secreted by these vesicles is released at ejaculation.

COWPER'S GLANDS (BULBOURETHRAL)

These two pea-sized glands secrete a clear fluid, known as "pre-cum." These secretions can contain living sperm; however, this happens chiefly when a male ejaculates for a second time without urinating between each ejaculation.

BEHIND THE BALLS AND INTO THE DUGOUT

The prostate gland has been mentioned with regards to its production of ejaculate. What wasn't highlighted, however, is the use of the prostate in producing what is often referred to as the male version of the G-Spot orgasm. It is therefore a crucial structure to locate when trying to "milk the prostate," an action that can produce these types of orgasms in many males. Take note of its location, and your finger nail length, as access occurs only from the rear. Refer to section Prostate Pleasure - Chapter 9 for more information on prostate milking during oral sex.

PERINEUM (AKA GOOCH/CHODA/TAINT)

The region between the anus and the scrotum (or the anus and the vulva in females). This area, when stroked appropriately, can produce stimulating results before, during, and after an orgasm.

ANUS AND RECTUM

The rectum is a more spacious area than the anus; therefore, most of the sensation generated during anal insertion (for both partners) derives from penetration of the anus itself, rather than the rectum. The anus is relatively tight and rich in nerves, which may be why anilingus and finger play can be an important addition for some when having a pleasurable oral experience.

"Clinton lied. A man might forget where he parks or where he lives, but he never forgets oral sex, no matter how bad it is." – Barbara Bush

Appendix B - Safety & Risks

Now, for the "not-very-fun-or-sexy-but-we-have-to-talk-about-it-anyways" section. There is no such thing as no-risk sexual contact however in the grand scheme of things, oral sex is on the low end of risky behaviours. That said, STI's (Sexually Transmitted Infections, formally known as STD's – Sexually Transmitted Diseases) that are passed from one partner to another during sex, can also be passed from one partner to another during oral sex. This means that, while moderately low, your chances of contracting something during oral sex is still a possibility, and dependent on where your partner's penis has ventured before meeting you.

Now that we've made things awkward for everyone, let's dive deeper and explore all the not-so-wonderful infections humans can share.

HIV

Using latex or polyurethane condoms, female condoms, or dental dams is an effective way to reduce your chances of contracting the virus when engaging in oral sex. Without protection, the risk of contracting HIV from oral sex increases if the person performing the act has cuts or sores in their mouth, if ejaculation takes place in the mouth, and if the individual receiving oral sex has any other sexually transmitted infections. The primary risk for HIV is for the person performing oral sex. Unless the partner has a significant amount of blood in their mouth - such as from dental surgery - oral sex is unlikely to expose the receiver to HIV.

It is important to keep in mind that a positive person's viral load will substantially affect the level of risk. For example, transmission from someone with an undetectable viral load (less than 40 copies per cubic milliliter in Canada / 200 copies internationally) is highly unlikely. The cause for concern is the 25% of people who are unaware of their infection (often claiming a negative status) or someone who is not on antiretroviral medication.

DID YOU KNOW?

Ejaculate-related sinus infection: it turns out, if you create a moderate vacuum around your partner's penis—and the timing of the ejaculate is just right (so that the head of the penis is at the back of your throat)— the suction can actually draw ejaculate up into one's sinus cavity, which in some, could cause a nasty sinus infection. Make sure to blow your nose; you'll most likely be fine (and have a good story to tell!).

HERPES

Although genital herpes is usually caused by the herpes simplex virus type 2 and oral herpes (also known as cold sores or fever blisters) is typically caused by herpes simplex virus type 1, both can be found on, and transmitted to/from the mouth, genitals, and other areas of the body. A common misconception is that if you already have one type of the virus you are immune to the other and sadly, this is not the case. You may be more resistant as your body already has the anti-bodies present, but transmission is still possible. It is important to be open and discuss with partners about the potential risks and take precautions as needed.

Condoms, female condoms, and dental dams can significantly reduce the risk of transmission. However since herpes can be present on body parts not covered by condoms—such as the scrotum, inner thigh, and buttocks—condoms are not a guarantee against exposure to the virus.

Another precaution that individuals can take is prescription anti-virals such as Valtrex and Zovirax that can help suppress the virus and reduce the incidence of outbreaks and transmitting the virus to others. Since you can spread the herpes virus to a partner even if you are not in an active outbreak phase, it is important to have open communication regarding your medical status, so both partners can make informed decisions.

HUMAN PAPILLOMAVIRUS VIRUS

As with herpes, it seems likely that the use of condoms or dental dams during oral sex should reduce the risk of infection from the Human Papillomavirus (HPV), which is linked to genital warts and various cancers. However, they will not necessarily eliminate it entirely since HPV spreads via skin-to-skin contact not through bodily fluids. It is possible to spread HPV through oral sex, and it is believed that HPV acquired while performing oral sex is a risk factor for oral and throat cancers.

Approximately 75% of sexually active adults will have an HPV infection at some point in their lives, although most people remain unaware of this and are able to clear the infection on their own.

DID YOU KNOW?

The majority of Canadians have at least one strain of the herpes virus in their system already, although a large proportion will never present with a symptom.

GONORRHEA

Gonorrhea is a bacterial infection that can be transmitted from throat to penis or penis to throat when oral sex is performed, and throat infections with gonorrhea are extremely difficult to treat. Also in most cases, the initial infection can have no symptoms. Condoms and dental dams should be extremely effective in preventing transmission of gonorrhea during oral sex as the usual site of transmission from the penis is the urethra.

CHLAMYDIA

It is possible to transmit Chlamydia during fellatio, and both the recipient and the person performing the act are at risk. Reported cases of Chlamydia rose from 2 to 207 per 100,000 persons between 1984 and 1997, and Chlamydia is now the most common of all reportable infectious diseases. As with Gonorrhea, condoms provide excellent protection from Chlamydia during oral sex.

SYPHILIS

Syphilis is easy to transmit via oral sex. Also, as it causes a break in the skin, it has been known to facilitate the spread of HIV as well. In fact, in some areas of the United States, oral sex has been shown to be responsible for as many as 15% of Syphilis cases. Although Syphilis can only be transmitted in the presence of symptoms, during the primary and secondary stages of the disease, the painless sores it causes are easy to miss.

HEPATITIS B

The research is inconclusive as to whether or not Hepatitis B can be transmitted via oral sex. Vaccination is a good idea in any case, and the Hepatitis B vaccine is currently available for all children and most adults.

Some other things to consider if you are planning on swallowing:

- Does your partner have a Sexually Transmitted Infection (STI) or a contagious blood borne disease?
- Has your partner had acute long-term exposure to poisons, heavy metals, radiation, or intravenous injections?
- Are you allergic to semen?
- Do you have cancerous tumours that could come into contact with concentrated ejaculate, or are sensitive to testosterone?

If you answered yes to any of these you may want to consider using condoms during oral sex to lower your risk level.

THE BOTTOM LINE

In summary, oral sex without condom use puts you at risk for numerous sexually transmitted infections, even if the risk may be low. If you perform unprotected oral sex on your sexual partners, you should mention it to your physician. Your doctor may want to check your throat when they are screening you for other STIs. Always be diligent, have you and your partner(s) tested, and maintain open communication with your sexual partners.

References

Aslan, Y., Atan, A., Aydın, A., Nalçacıoğlu, V., Tuncel, A., & Kadıoğlu, A. (2011). *Penile length and somatometric parameters: A study in healthy young Turkish men.* Asian Journal of Andrology, 13, 339-341. DOI:10.1038/aja.2010.109

Auslander, B., Rosenthal, S. Fortenberry, D., Biro, F., Bernstein, D., & Zimet, G. (2007). *Predictors of sexual satisfaction in an adolescent and college population.* Journal of Pediatric and Adolescent Gynecology, 20(1), 25-28. DOI:http://dx.doi.org/10.1016/j.jpag.2006.10.006

Boskey, E. (2013, August 20). *Is Oral Sex Safe Sex?* Retrieved September 13, 2013, from http://std.about.com/od/riskfactorsforstds/a/oralsexsafesex.htm

Bridges, S., Lease, S., & Ellison, C. (2004). *Predicting sexual satisfaction in women: Implications for counselor education and training.* Journal of Counseling & Development, 82(2), 158-166. DOI: 10.1002/j.1556-6678.2004.tb00297.x

Buzzell, T. (2005). *Demographic characteristics of persons using pornography in three technological contexts.* Sexuality & Culture, 9(1), 28-48. DOI:10.1007/BF02908761

Byers, S., Demmon, S., & Lawrance, K. (1998). *Sexual satisfaction within dating relationships: A test of the interpersonal exchange model of sexual satisfaction.* Journal of Social and Personal Relationships, 7(2), 227–245. DOI:10.5964/ijpr.v7i2.141

Cerny, J., & Janssen, E. (2011). *Patterns of sexual arousal in homosexual, bisexual, and heterosexual men.* Archives of Sexual Behavior, 40(4), 687-697. DOI:10.1007/s10508-011-9746-0

Chandra, A., Mosher, W. D., Copen, C., & Sionean, C. (2011). *Sexual behavior, sexual attraction, and sexual identity in the United States.* Data from the 2006–2008 national survey of family growth. National Health Statistics Reports: Centers for Disease Control and Prevention, 36. Retrieved March 12, 2013, from http://www.ncbi.nlm.nih.gov/pubmed/21560887

Cooper, A., Scherer, C., Boies, S., & Gordon, B. (1999). *Sexuality on the Internet: From sexual exploration to pathological expression.* Professional Psychology: Research and Practice, 30(2), 154-164. DOI: 10.1037/0735-7028.30.2.154

Davis, C., Blank, J., Lin, H., & Bonillas, C. (1996). *Characteristics of vibrator use among women.* Journal of Sex Research, 33(4), 313-320. DOI:10.1080/00224499609551848

Delacoste, F. (1987). *Sex work: Writings by women in the sex industry.* Pittsburgh, Pa.: Cleis Press.

Edwards, J. N. and A. Booth (1994). *Sexuality, marriage, and well-being: The middle years. Sexuality across the life course.* The John D. and Catherine T. MacArthur Foundation series on mental health and development: Studies on successful midlife development. A. S. E. Rossi. Chicago, The University of Chicago Press: 233-259

Edwards, S., & Carne, C. (1998). *Oral sex and transmission of non-viral STIs.* Sexually Transmitted Infections, 74(2), 95-100. DOI: 10.1136/sti.74.2.95

Ernulf, K., & Innala, S. (1995). *Sexual bondage: A review and unobtrusive investigation.* Archives of Sexual Behavior, 24(6), 631-654. DOI:10.1007/BF01542185

Facts on American Teens' Sexual and Reproductive Health (2010). Alan Guttmacher Institute. New York: AGI. www.guttmacher.org/pubs/FB-ATSRH.pdf

Festinger, L. (1954). *A theory of social comparison processes.* Human Relations, 7, 117-140. DOI: 10.1177/001872675400700202

Fox, K. (2006). *The smell report.* Social Issues Research Center. Retrieved March 11, 2013, from http://www.sirc.org/publik/smell.pdf

Geddes, D. (1954). *An analysis of the Kinsey reports on sexual behavior in the human male and female.* New York: Dutton.

Glasier, A., Gülmezoglu, A., Schmid, G., Moreno, C., & Van Look, P. (2006). *Sexual and reproductive health: A matter of life and death.* The Lancet, 368(9547), 1595-1607. DOI:http://dx.doi.org/10.1016/S0140-6736(06)69478-6

Holmberg, D., & Blair, K. L. (2009). *Sexual desire, communication, satisfaction, and preferences of men and women in same-sex versus mixed-sex relationships.* Journal of Sex Research, 46(1), 57-66. DOI:10.1080/00224490802645294

Hummel, C. L. (2010). *Impact of sexual frequency on sexual satisfaction, relationship satisfaction, and self-esteem.* Unpublished master's thesis, Adler University, Vancouver, British Columbia.

Janus, S., & Janus, C. (1993). *The Janus report on sexual behavior.* New York: John Wiley.

Joannides, P. (2009). *Guide to getting it on: For adults of all ages.* Waldport, Oregon: Goofy Foot Press.

Kent, C., Chaw, J., Wong, W., Liska, S., Gibson, S., Hubbard, G., & Klausner, J. (2005). *Prevalence of rectal, urethral, and pharyngeal chlamydia and gonorrhea detected in 2 clinical settings among men who have sex with men:* San Francisco, California, 2003. Clinical Infectious Diseases, 41(1), 67-74. DOI:10.1089/apc.2008.0277

Kohl, J., & Francoeur, R. (1995). *The scent of eros: Mysteries of odor in human sexuality.* New York: Continuum.

Kreimer, A., Alberg, A., Daniel, R., Gravitt, P., Viscidi, R., Garrett, E., . . . Gillison, M. (2004). *Oral human papillomavirus infection in adults is associated with sexual behavior and HIV serostatus.* The Journal of Infectious Diseases, 189(4), 686-698. DOI:10.1086/381504

Lafferty, W., Downey, L., Celum, C., & Wald, A. (2000). H*erpes simplex virus type 1 as a cause of genital herpes: Impact on surveillance and prevention.* The Journal of Infectious Diseases, 181(4), 1454-1457. DOI:10.1086/315395

Lambert, D. (2005). *The secret sex lives of animals.* New York: Sterling Pub.

Leitenberg, H., & Henning, K. (1996). *Sexual fantasy.* Psychological Bulletin, 117(3), 469-496. DOI:http://dx.doi. org/10.1037/0033-2909.117.3.469

LeVay, S., & Valente, S. (2002). *Human sexuality.* Sunderland, Mass.: Sinauer Associates.

Masters, W., & Johnson, V. (1966). *Human sexual response.* Boston: Little, Brown and Company.

McCary, J. (1967). *Human sexuality: Physiological and psychological factors of sexual behavior.* New York: Van Nostrand Reinhold.

Meston, C. M., & Buss, D. M. (2007). *Why humans have sex.* Archives of Sexual Behaviour, 36, 477-507. DOI: 10.1007/s10508-007-9175-2

Paget, L. (1999). *How to be a great lover: Girlfriend-to-girlfriend totally explicit techniques that will blow his mind*. New York: Broadway Books.

Papp, J., Ahrens, K., Phillips, C., Kent, C., Philip, S., & Klausner, J. (2007). *The use and performance of oral–throat rinses to detect pharyngeal Neisseria gonorrhoeae and Chlamydia trachomatis infections*. Diagnostic Microbiology and Infectious Disease, 59, 259–264. DOI:http://dx.doi.org/10.1016/j.diagmicrobio.2007.05.010

Petermana T. A., & Furnessa, B.W. (2007). *The resurgence of syphilis among men who have sex with men*. Current Opinions in Infectious Diseases, 20(1), 54–59. DOI:10.1097/QCO.0b013e32801158cc

Robinson, B. E., Bockting, W. O, & Harrell, T. (2002). *Masturbation and sexual health: An exploratory study of low-income african-american women*. Journal of Psychology and Human Sexuality, 14(2/3), 85-102. DOI:10.1300/J056v14n02_06

Schiavi, R., Derogatis, L., Kuriansky, J., O'connor, D., & Sharpe, L. (2008). *The assessment of sexual function and marital interaction*. Journal of Sex & Marital Therapy, 169-224. DOI:10.1080/00926237908403730

Sex and America's Teenagers (1994). Alan Guttmacher Institute. New York: AGI. www.guttmacher.org/pubs/archive/SaAT.pdf

Sexual and Reproductive Health: Women and Men (2002). Alan Guttmacher Institute. New York: AGI. www.guttmacher.org/pubs/fb_10-02.html

Sexually Transmitted Diseases in America: How Many Cases and at What Cost? (1998). Kaiser Family Foundation, American Social Health Association. Retrieved April 14, 2013, from http://www.kff.org/content/archive/1445/std_rep.pdf

Sexual health—a new focus for WHO. Progress in Sexual and Reproductive Health Research. (2004). World Health Organization Report, www.who.int/hrp/publications/progress67.pdf

Sherrow, V. (2001). *For Appearance's Sake: The Historical Encyclopedia of Good Looks, Beauty, and Grooming.* Connecticut: Greenwood Publishing. DOI:10.1336/1573562041

Stephen, I., & Mckeegan, A. (2010). *Lip colour affects perceived sex typicality and attractiveness of human faces.* Perception, 39(8) 1104-1110. DOI:10.1068/p6730

Tan, M., Jones, G., Zhu, G., Ye, J., Hong, T., Zhou, S., . . . Hosken, D. (2009). *Fellatio by Fruit Bats Prolongs Copulation Time.* PLoS ONE 4(10), E7595-E7595. DOI:10.1371/journal.pone.0007595

Transmission of Primary and Secondary Syphilis by Oral Sex --- Chicago, Illinois, 1998--2002. (2004, October 22). Morbidity and Mortality Weekly Report, 966-968.

VanYperen, N. W., & Buunk, B. P. (1991). *Sex-role attitudes, social comparisons, and satisfaction with relationships.* Social Psychology Quarterly, 54(2), 169-180. Article retrieved from: http://www.jstor.org/stable/2786934

Viral Hepatitis, STD and TB Prevention. Centres for Disease Control and Prevention. National Centre for HIV/AIDS, (2013, March 17\)Retrieved April 17, 2015 from http://www.cdc.gov/nchhstp/Default.htm

Wellings, K. (1995). *The Social Organization of Sexuality: Sexual Practices in the United States; Sex in America: A Definitive Survey.* BMJ, 310, 540. DOI:http://dx.doi.org/10.1136/bmj.310.6978.540

White, J. B., Langer, E. J., Yariv, L., & Welch, J. C. (2006). *Frequent social comparisons and destructive emotions and behaviors: The dark side of social comparison.* Journal of Adult Development, 13(1), 36-44. DOI:10.1007/s10804-006-9005-0

Winston, M. (1987). *The biology of the honey bee.* Cambridge, Mass.: Harvard University Press.

Zurbriggen, E. L., & Yost, M. R. (2004). *Power, desire, and pleasure in sexual fantasies.* Journal of Sex Research, 41(3), 288-300. DOI:10.1080/00224490409552236

About the Authors

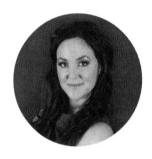

DR. TEESHA MORGAN

Psychotherapist, Sexologist, TEDx Speaker & Media Personality

Dr. Teesha Morgan is a Sex Therapist and Couples Counsellor whose background includes a Doctorate in Human Sexuality, a Master of Arts in Counselling Psychology specializing in Sex Therapy, and a Bachelors of Science – Major in Psychology, Additionally, Dr. Morgan holds an Associate in Sex Education and Clinical Sexology certificate, making her one of the few Sex Therapists & Clinical Sexologists in Canada. Teesha is also the Co-Founder of The Westland Academy of Clinical Sex Therapy.

www.TeeshaMorgan.com

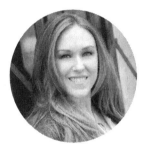

CONSTANCE LYNN HUMMEL, MA

Psychotherapist, Leadership Coach, Clinical Supervisor, Speaker

Constance holds a Master of Arts in Counselling Psychology, and in her clinical practice she specializes in Relationships, Sex Therapy, and Addictions. Her graduate research explored the impact that sexual frequency has on sexual and relationship satisfaction, as well as self-esteem in long-term relationships. Additionally she has extensive training in the Gottman Couples Therapy Method and Emotion Focused Therapy for Couples. Constance is also the Co-Founder of The Westland Academy of Clinical Sex Therapy.

www.ConstanceLynn.com

Made in the USA
San Bernardino, CA
29 October 2017